The Peace of Mind Playlist

Strategies and songs to help quieten your inner critic

Paul Parry

Edited by Rachel Kenny

Typesetting by Charlotte Mouncey www.bookstyle.co.uk

Cover design by Jonathan Cooksley

Illustrations by Lizzie Knott

The Peace of Mind Playlist – Strategies and songs to help quieten your inner critic

thepeaceofmindplaylist.com

paulparry.com

For book updates, premium content and exclusive offers, join my mailing list at TPoMP.com

ISBN 978-1-8384473-0-4

Disclaimer:

The information presented in this book should not be treated as a substitute for qualified medical advice. Neither the author nor the publisher can be held responsible for any loss or claim arising out of the use, or misuse, of the suggestions made or the failure to take medical advice.

If you're in the UK and you or someone else is in danger, call 999 or go to A&E now. If you need help urgently for your mental health, but it's not an emergency, call the NHS on 111 or visit 111.nhs.uk. Your mental health is as important as your physical health. You will not be wasting anyone's time. Visit this NHS website for urgent support: nhs.uk/every-mind-matters/urgent-support.

For confidential support on suicide matters in the UK, call the Samaritans on 116 123 or visit samaritans.org for more ways to contact them.

In the USA, call the 988 Suicide & Crisis Lifeline on 988 or visit 988lifeline.org.

For my mum, who always gave me peace of mind.

Contents

Preface: Start

"You can't get rid of what you carry around in your metaphorical backpack. All you can do is take that pack off, look inside and rearrange it so it doesn't mess up other parts of your life, like your relationships or your children." – Huey Morgan

I see a former colleague's post on LinkedIn. It's the summer of 2022, and the post is about people who work away from home for weeks at a time at big sports events, like I occasionally do, and how some of those people sometimes struggle with what's going on inside their heads. That post really resonates with me. I think, "I want to say things like that on platforms like this, so why don't I?"

I consider how I'd like to curb my tendency to overthink, rein in my penchant for impostor syndrome, and stem the tide of self-critical thought which I've been prone to for as long as I can remember. A tendency, which, in 2022, routinely stumbled into my working day with the discretion of a drunk tripping over a chair leg while carrying a tray of eggs.

On Spotify, I scroll through the playlists I put together every year to help me remember the funny, beautiful and important moments that occurred during a particular set of 12 months.

And now I watch from afar as a bloke I've never met builds a community project for men's mental health, aiming to break the stigma of this topic and talk openly about it. I think:

"That's brilliant. I want to do something like that for people like that."

The Peace of Mind Playlist is my attempt to bring those things together, primarily for blokes over 30. A stab at combining personal stories with some of the science – in plain English, mind – that drives the human brain. Strategies to help quieten your inner critic. And a varied, accompanying playlist, featuring 49 tracks, old and new, that spans the moods. A new, varied playlist for people who like new, varied playlists.

Featured artists include:

The Jam / The Saints / The Streets / David Bowie / FPI Project / Stardust / Reverend And The Makers / Fatboy Slim / Blu DeTiger / Kool & The Gang / Gerry Rafferty / Laurent Garnier / The Primitives / Bjork / The Stranglers / Elvis / Portishead / Depeche Mode / Massive Attack / Half Man Half Biscuit / Bob Marley & The Wailers / Red Hot Chili Peppers / Ian Dury & The Blockheads / Beastie Boys / The Beatles / JJ Cale / Slacker / Fun Boy Three / Hot Chip / The Clash / Jess Glynne / Soft Cell / Pink Floyd / The Smiths / Leftfield / Kristine W / Death of Guitar Pop / Pantera / Lane 8 / Selena Gomez / Jane's Addiction / The Ting Tings / Oasis / The Damned / Groove Armada / Cast / Etta James

The first part of the book (five songs) offers a bit more context to the pages that follow. Part 2 (seven songs) looks at getting started, while Part 3 (15 songs) presents science and scenarios. Part 4 (21 songs) is where you'll find the meat (or meat substitute if you're vegan). This is where the 18 strategies are explained. Accessible mental health support for blokes who could do with accessible mental health support.

The book's premise explores two key areas of our brain that work differently. One is primal, the other evolved more recently and is more rational. By the time you get to Part 4, you'll hopefully – if I've done my job well – have a clear understanding of how these two areas of the brain function and can make us feel. With this knowledge, Part 4's strategies can then be used more effectively, and reinforced by music.

The power of the playlist should not be underestimated. Playlists are handy, shareable and powerful. They can give us something special, like old photos. They can rekindle memories of a time, a place or a loved one. And they can help someone going through a tough time remember some useful, proven strategies to alleviate the stress a little. Playlists can surprise, energise or remind. Press play for peace of mind.

I often wonder whether *The Peace of Mind Playlist,* which you'll find on Spotify (I'll give you the link later), should be focused on one or two genres, such as house, or ska and 2 Tone. In the end, I adopted the premise of the playlists I create for every year: the memories are mixed, the moments mingle, and so the music varies. Just like life. Music, with all its different moods, comforts us, soothes us, reassures us like an old friend. It can spur us into action, invigorate or relax us. Music can help us remember the things that lead to peace of mind.

So who am I?

I'm Paul Parry – friends call me Pazza – a middle-aged bald bloke who works in sport (basically, I'm very similar to Pep Guardiola when you think about it, and I've been to Barcelona, Munich and Manchester). A freelancer, for early clients I built and hosted websites, blogged or wrote content for search engine optimisation (SEO). Like lots of us, I've done a few things over the years to pay the bills, and those are just a few of them. These days, I'm a sub-editor, an operations manager, and I'm one of the three partners behind Amp Media, which is a content agency working primarily with international sports organisations. That's a lot of sport, which I love just as much as I love music, and probably why sport and athletes feature quite heavily in these pages. *The Peace of Mind Playlist* is my fourth self-published book. The others are *Pazzabaijan* (2015), *Mr Lizard* (2017), and *Working Remotely – How to promote your internet-based business* (2020).

Why should you listen to me?

Like Scott Johnson, I'm a bloke trying to break the stigma of men's mental health by encouraging conversation on this topic. And, like Kate Lamb, my former colleague who posted something inspiring on LinkedIn I refer to later, I want to say things on public platforms that will hopefully reach and help people who sometimes struggle with what's going on inside their heads.

I'm not a doctor. I'm not qualified in these things. But I have been quite good at tying myself in mental knots, worrying unnecessarily and overthinking my overthinking. And in the two years since the Beijing 2022 Olympic Winter Games, I've learned how to identify, understand and manage this kind of thinking and improve my life with much more peace of mind. In the process of producing *The Peace of Mind Playlist*, I reckon I've reduced my negative or unhelpful thinking by as much as 90%. I'd like nothing more now than to help other people – *you*, maybe – to do something similar, to enjoy more peace of mind by using a proven set of strategies and a hand-picked playlist. Press play for peace of mind – but remember: you can't silence your inner critic merely by turning up the volume. The songs in that playlist can help in isolation but are best served in combination with their corresponding strategies in the book. Read or listen to the book (an audio version will be available only to a select bunch – and you're virtually in already), and enjoy the playlist as the songs remind you of a particular story or strategy or scientific fact.

Finally, I must emphasise that the information presented in this book should not be treated as a substitute for qualified medical advice. If you're in the UK and you or someone else is in danger, call 999 or go to A&E now. If you need help urgently for your mental health, but it's not an emergency, call the NHS on 111 or visit 111.nhs.uk. Your mental health is as important as your physical health. You will not be wasting anyone's time.

- *The Peace of Mind Playlist* is the result of two years of focused research and about 17 years of casual research – books and blog posts I've read, podcasts I've listened to, therapy sessions I've babbled my way through and so on.

- If you like books such as *The Chimp Paradox, Why Has Nobody Told Me This Before?* or *Think Like A Monk,* you might enjoy *The Peace of Mind Playlist.*

- No need to carry the book around with you for backup – *The Peace of Mind Playlist* via Spotify on your phone will do just fine.

- So, are you in?

For updates on the book, exclusive content and to listen to the playlist, head to:

thepeaceofmindplaylist.com

PART 1: introduction

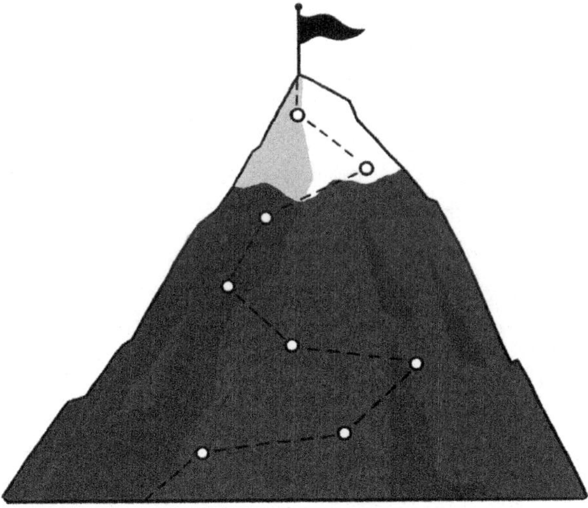

I'm Stranded

A head-shaped horrorbox

Early in 2022, I spent a couple of months in Beijing at the winter Olympics. I'm neither a figure skater nor one of those lunatics who flings themselves down a mountain head-first on a tea tray in a quest for skeleton gold. No, I was covering the Games as a journalist.

And while there is pressure to do a good job, there is not the need to perform at my best in front of millions of people around the world regardless of how I feel, which I'm sure makes life slightly easier to cope with when you're not quite feeling all together up top, when something hard to articulate makes your head feel a bit all over the place.

The restrictions within restrictions intended to limit the spread of Covid everyone at those Olympics faced – translucent sheets covering hotel windows, and polystyrene boards dividing people either side of dining tables, for example – didn't help me when I was already feeling low or emotionally drained, or both. Nor, I suspect, did they help to curb the possible spread of Covid, but that's another debate.

I've worked away from home at events for weeks on end a few times, including at the Rugby World Cup, Wimbledon, European Games, European Championships and Global Esports Games, as well as winter, summer and youth Olympics.

Occasionally while away, I've worried, felt nervous or carried on despite feeling like an impostor. I've felt anxious or prone to homesickness. But I am exceptionally good at keeping on top of the washing. I'll carefully observe the chief explorer of the group as he enters the office one morning having sussed out the location and operation of the laundry facilities we've been provided with. I'll go soon after, and come back feeling more than a little smug, like I've just fixed the global economy with a speech at the UN.

In Beijing, negative feelings got the better of me a lot of the time. I felt stranded, I couldn't think clearly and I wasn't getting any comfort from my usual daily rituals like a morning run, coffee or calls home.

What was described as the closed loop, the system designed to protect anyone who was working at the Olympics in any capacity from contracting Covid by preventing us from having any contact with the outside world, was eroding my cheerfulness. Inside my head, unhelpful and negative thoughts were rampant and often piled up on top of one another, like a torrent flowing into a bigger torrent.

While everyone around me seemed to be coping well, I was longing for home and told myself and others "Not long now" when they and I knew we still had weeks to go.

I felt self-doubt, worry or anxiety triggered by everyday things such as a phone ringing or needing to make basic amendments to a spreadsheet, and less everyday things including my 50th birthday, which my brilliant and generous colleagues helped me to celebrate shortly before the Paralympics started.

One day, I looked out of my 12th-floor hotel room window, understanding properly for the first time why a person might feel like flinging themselves from such a height. I didn't feel that urge – falling out of my kingsize bed on to a soft carpet a couple of weeks earlier was scary enough – but I did understand how someone might get there.

I struggled psychologically more in Beijing during those two months than at any other time or in any other place in my life.

Turn The Page

Deciding to improve resilience

I'm someone who's often been held back by thinking I'm not worthy, or that I'm a pain in the backside, or only in my post until I get found out and they put me on the first bus home. Beijing was simply the latest in a long list of experiences I'd grappled with. Because of my struggles, while I'm not a neuroscientist, psychiatrist, psychotherapist or doctor myself, I occasionally absorb the knowledge doctors, neuroscientists, psychiatrists and psychotherapists share to help people with common problems such as nervousness, worry, anxiety, impostor syndrome and homesickness. I used that insight to help me write a book in 2017, *Mr Lizard,* in which I explored experts' knowledge of these issues and potential solutions to reduce or even eliminate the detrimental impact they can have in everyday life.

Originally intended for teenagers, primarily because I have children who were that age at the time (and I occasionally still feel like one), the Mr Lizard concept was designed to help readers understand our prehistoric cognitive tendencies. I wanted to highlight and explore the internal battle that goes on all the time between our ears. In the blue corner, our more rational, 'human' thought processes. In the red, from Waybackwhen and representing our prehistoric instincts, including emotion, Mr Lizard.

I started thinking about writing this book you hold in your hands when I returned home from Beijing with a suitcase full of clean, beautifully smelling laundry and a compulsion to start thinking differently. I wanted to continue working at sports events. I knew I deserved to enjoy working at sports events, and working at them helps to pay my bills, but it was time to get serious, to turn the page psychologically.

I started by doing a lot of research into proven solutions to help relieve the unhelpful thoughts which have had a negative effect on my life and that of many others, then I began implementing a select few of them. This book – which expands on the themes in *Mr Lizard* – is the culmination of that research.

We kick off with a basic examination of what's inside our heads, backed up by science and explained in plain English. This is a book with self-awareness, reframing and metacognition – thinking about thinking – at its core. You don't need to be any particular type of person to benefit from what I've learned and share here.

Then we move on to a set of 18 evidence-based strategies and practical solutions to better manage negative and hindering patterns of thought, and challenging situations, that crop up every day, when our rational thinking can feel like it's been hijacked by the emotional part of the brain, the amygdala. I've drawn these from a number of resources – books, films, apps, radio interviews, coaching, courses, blind intuition, drunken instincts, and songs. Think of these strategies as tools in a box, each designed to serve a specific purpose. I demonstrate how they can be employed using stories from my own life and hypothetical scenarios.

The strategies I explain in this book are the solid resource I (and you, I hope) can turn to when times are tough. In those times, it's worth remembering too that, just like clear blue sky, the 'real you' is always there, even when your lizard brain and emotions skew your perception of events or who you are.

Finally, this book is neither therapy nor individual advice. It is not an alternative to treatment of serious psychological conditions such as depression, addiction, suicidal tendencies or post-traumatic stress disorder.

Before we move on, let me leave you with the wise words of the psychotherapist and author of *How To Be Your Own Therapist*, Owen O'Kane: "If you're low and you're really struggling and things are not good, (remember) it's not a permanent state and it doesn't have to be a permanent state. Things can improve and things do improve."

Changes

Making change happen

For many years, I worked in transmission in London's TV industry. This meant I had to sit and watch telly for 12 hours at a time (day or night) and make sure everyone else who was watching the output I was looking after saw the correct pictures and not colour bars, a black screen or Premier League football by accident. That last one took a bit of explaining, but I'll leave that for another time.

The programming I had to watch included all sorts: police officers, cartoons, paranormal characters called Sam, and infomercials – 30-minute, information-based commercials, often selling mops or blenders or maybe toy giraffes. I must admit I usually stopped watching about 30 seconds in. I could monitor my channels without actually watching every minute of output.

One infomercial I did pay some attention to was called *Get The Edge*. It promoted a self-help product of the same name which had been created by the author and coach Tony Robbins. I hadn't heard of him at the time, and used to sit there, feeling half-dead at five in the morning at the tail-end of a 12-hour night shift, microwave curry box still on the desk next to a printed copy of the transmission schedule, taking in what Mr Robbins had to say.

One of the ideas I learned from this infomercial was that while change in our lives is automatic, progress is not. For example, we can't control friends or bosses moving away, tax increases or the death of a loved one. Changes such as these just happen whether we like them or not. Actually making progress in our lives – maybe through academic achievement, or applying for a particular job or deciding to attend a specific event which could open doors for us – tends to occur as a result of decisions we make. The idea that Robbins was explaining in his infomercial led me to study change in more detail, both how to manage it and how to make it happen.

Later, I came across *Switch: How to change things when change is hard*. Its authors, the brothers Chip and Dan Heath, discuss change in organisations, communities and our lives – "changes," as they put it, "that matter to you, whether your interest is in changing the world or changing your waistline".

In the book, they talk about change such as improving a decades-old medical practice that was endangering patients, a technique for overcoming the dread of housework, and transforming an apathetic customer-support team into an enthused and effective operation. Change, they suggest, often fails because the primitive side of our brain, what they call the Elephant and I call the Lizard, and our rational side – the Rider/human – can't co-operate for long enough to effect the desired switch.

The authors also suggest change fails because our environment, what they call the Path, isn't conducive. What might be perceived as a 'people problem' is often a 'situation problem'. For example, a local council might be faced with people routinely driving too fast along a particular road within that local authority's jurisdiction. The council understands that in order to reduce the number of accidents on that particular stretch of road, speeding drivers must slow down. But rather than regarding those drivers and their behaviour as the problem – why won't they slow down? – and recognising that changing their habits is a persistent headache, the council might instead consider adjusting the situation in order to solve the problem: in this case, the road, where the issue actually lies.

Speeding drivers can easily be encouraged to slow down and proceed more cautiously with the installation of traffic lights, clearer lane markings, speed cameras, humps in the road and traffic islands to prevent dangerous overtaking. In other words, drivers will slow down when their environment tells them or forces them to.

Tweaking the environment – the Path – is about making the wrong behaviours harder and the better action easier.

To make change happen, the Chip brothers say we must (1) direct the Rider, (2) motivate the Elephant and (3) shape the Path.

1) Direct your Rider/human by creating a clear vision of the outcome you seek, and listing the actions and tactics required to get there.

2) Strong feelings, such as needing to change, and hope, motivate Elephants and Lizards. Therefore, the Heath brothers write, it pays to engineer some

early successes or quick wins, which bring hope (Elephants and Lizards often hate doing things with no immediate pay-off).

3) Shaping the Path means removing hurdles or tweaking your environment to allow change to happen as easily as possible.

In 2013, I completed the London marathon. It took a while, and I refused to let being overtaken by a Womble throw me off my stride. When training for the big day, and needing to get in the habit of running regularly, I'd lay out my kit the night before an early-morning run, just to make it as easy as possible to leave the house. I'd learned that by making the right thing to do the easy thing to do, I stood more of a chance of actually getting out to train as I'd intended.

Everybody (All Over the World)

We're not alone

Seven-time Wimbledon champion Novak Djokovic said after winning his quarter-final in 2022:

"Even though I've played tennis on the big stage for 20 years now, I go through the same doubtful moments as anybody else. The inner fight is always the biggest fight on the court and off the court, so trying to win that internal fight is a big challenge.

"Once you do that, I feel like external circumstances are more likely to go in your favour."

A LinkedIn post I read a few weeks later, shortly after the 2022 Commonwealth Games, confirmed that this "inner fight" is common to us all. The post, written by Kate Lamb, a friend, former colleague and a brilliant broadcast engineer, is reproduced with her kind permission and lightly edited for additional clarity:

"So here I am on the last day of the Commonwealth Games. I'm sitting in my hotel room writing this and reflecting on the past three weeks.

"I have worked on major events in the past but one thing really hit me this time. Three weeks away from family and friends, submerged in work that we all love to do at an event that we all want to be part of with colleagues who are great – but yet it has its downsides.

"I met many people – colleagues – who are really struggling. Two or three weeks away from home in a broadcasting bubble places us in a unique mindspace. It affords us time to reflect on life, it brings opportunities to meet new people and make new connections and reassess our life goals. Any worries or concerns can come to the fore of our minds and as a result can feel overwhelming.

"This major event has seen me hold the hand of a colleague as he cried. I have listened and supported other colleagues as best I can as they spoke of their private and professional worries.

"I can't help feeling that there's a great opportunity that is being missed here. I would love to see a safe, welcoming space at a major event, where colleagues can sit and talk and open up about any worries or problems they are experiencing. Maybe in partnership with a charity like Mind or The Film and TV Charity where if necessary people can be signposted to receive help.

"In my mind I imagine a chill-out room in the International Broadcast Centre (IBC) where people can sit and have a coffee in comfortable surroundings with colleagues – run by volunteers.

"Here at the IBC for the Commonwealth Games, I saw lounge spaces that were exclusive corporate spaces for sponsors, clients and execs to gather and network – and that's all part of the event. That's fine – but what about the rest of the workforce who are living in hotel rooms for three weeks? Some might be at crisis point.

"Time away from home for some may also be respite from issues that they may not be able to chat about over a pint at the bar with colleagues – this time away may be a golden opportunity for them to reach out to someone for help or guidance in how to cope when the event is over and the de-rig done.

"Please – I would love to hear what others think about this – would you like to see a chill-out space at a major event for colleagues? Would you like to know that there is someone there to talk to who will listen – even if you just want to chat about how much you are missing home? Let's open up the conversation."

Djokovic, it turns out – with all his success on the tennis court – is just like those of us who might not be sporting greats in that he too must deal with the battle between his ears. Where he differs – much like the snooker player Ronnie O'Sullivan, who is also a seven-time world champion and has also had internal battles to manage at and away from the snooker table – lies perhaps in his ability to identify what's happening and where he might be going wrong from a psychological perspective, clearly understanding why this is a factor precisely when he needs to, and finding a way to manage "doubtful moments" in order to stand a greater chance of achieving the desired outcome.

If legends of sport can identify, understand and manage difficult moments when competing for a world title in front of a huge global audience, it gives me hope that the rest of us can help ourselves out of a hole just when we need to as well. It's helpful then to have a few strategies and methods we can turn to.

Shaping the Path doesn't have to be physical; it can be psychological too (hence the expression 'get out of your own way'). We can all at least try to build mental resilience by using proven strategies which are designed to help us in sticky moments, even if the aim is to feel more comfortable in an office environment rather than to win a world title.

Music Sounds Better With You

Using music

Music taps into our emotions like nothing else, engaging and inspiring both on an individual level and en masse. The Abbey Road Institute, which trains music producers and sound engineers, says the music lots of us relate to acts as an extension of ourselves, and that it's a form of expression. Music, the institute says, tells a story, serving as a "social glue" and binding us in a way that language rarely does.

I believe in the power of music to relax, energise, and create memories, a sense of community and connection. I believe that hearing a familiar song for the first time in ages feels like meeting up with an old friend, and listening to a curated playlist is a good way to enjoy music.

This is why each chapter in this book, just as in *Mr Lizard*, shares its title with a song. While not every title is mentioned in the chapter that comes after it, the sentiment of each song title does at least match that of the words which follow.

This is significant not just because of a fondness for the music I've chosen. It's also because hearing the songs repeatedly on an easily accessible playlist might help us remember the corresponding idea and reduce the time wasted dwelling on negative or unhelpful thoughts.

Read the book, listen to the playlist – find it at thepeaceofmindplaylist.com – and remember the strategies that can help you achieve more peace of mind. The strategies in this book, and this playlist, have helped me reduce overthinking by what feels like 90%, and more comfortably navigate one of the most challenging events in my life, which we'll get to later.

PART 2: getting started

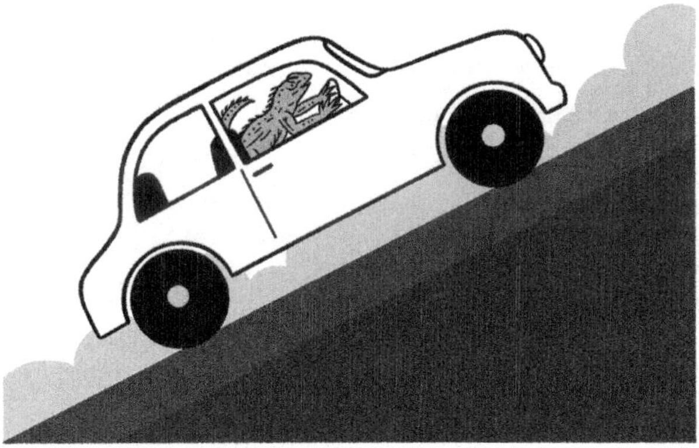

The State of Things

Bear Grylls is right

In October 2023, Matthew Taylor, the chief executive of the NHS Confederation, described the state of mental healthcare in England as a "national emergency". Fourteen months earlier, Taylor's colleague Sean Duggan, chief executive of the NHS Confederation's Mental Health Network, said: "Even before the pandemic, there had been growing levels of need for mental health services and this has been exacerbated by the impacts of the pandemic.

"Projections show 10 million people in England – including 1.5 million children and teenagers – will need new or additional support for their mental health over the next three to five years."

So, what is going on?

The world's favourite adventurer seems to know, at least in the case of the children and teenagers. A month after Sean Duggan's comments, Bear Grylls told *The Times*:

"There's such a gulf between school and life. The ill-equipping of young people is why we're experiencing an anxiety pandemic. It's very hard for young people. I don't think it's ever been harder because so much is coming at them all at the same time at a million miles an hour.

"You're confronted with everything from drugs, addiction stuff, to social media, to peer pressure, to the competitive world of getting a job, to lockdown, to environmental concerns, to Ukraine."

Young people in particular are having to deal with so much but without the necessary support and, in addition, they're at a biological disadvantage: the part of the human brain which enables rational thinking and suppresses our most brutal and least pleasant animalistic urges, the prefrontal cortex, doesn't fully develop until well after adolescence.

Teenagers' brains are more sensory than cognitive – in other words, they feel more than they think. Although the human brain matures in size during adolescence, important developments within the prefrontal cortex and other regions occur well into our 20s, and research suggests that most human brains take about 25 years to develop, with rates varying among individuals and among men and women – connections in the brain generally become streamlined earlier in girls than in boys.

Right Here, Right Now

It's up to us

Based on what I've seen, heard, read and experienced, I believe we urgently need more and better education on mental health. But successive UK governments have not been up to the job so it's looking like the rest of us might have to step up.

We need effective solutions to alleviate the anxieties which so many of us face daily. We need new skills. We need to cultivate self-awareness. We need to better understand how, why and when we think as rational humans and how, why and when we're more likely to react like the apes we're related to. We need insight on how this paradox can often leave us feeling, and knowledge of what we can do to mitigate those consequences in the face of multiple challenges, both online and in the physical world.

Instead of trying to cure and failing miserably, let's aim to prevent our mental health from cracking – or even merely creaking. We need something we can turn to when we need to restore stability or when we're having a bad day and feeling stranded.

What we need is a set of evidence-based strategies and practical solutions to help quieten our inner critics, things we can each do to try to manage negative and hindering patterns of thought, and challenging situations.

Figure It Out

Learn and progress

Curb negative thinking. Easier said than done, I hear you say. So, what do you do when popular advice such as "Too much analysis causes paralysis" or "Others may press your buttons but it's up to you what comes up on the screen" just doesn't cut it? When, like I've been in the past, you're overly worried about saying the wrong thing and upsetting someone, or not adequately doing the job you've been hired to do, or no one finding any of your jokes even remotely funny – all examples of what Dr Pippa Grange, who's a psychologist for elite sportsmen and women and the author of *Fear Less,* describes as 'not-good-enough' fear rather than 'in-the-moment' fear.

Some people turn to social media to learn strategies for dealing with anxiety and stress. Others seek advice from friends, family or a professional. I tend to lean on films, apps, radio interviews, coaching or courses. Or I'll read books. Slowly.

There's more information available than can ever be learned so you need to carefully select the appropriate tools for *you* that will prevent you from overthinking past events, feeling nervous when a phone rings, fearing sneezing in the office (more on that – aaa, achew – later) or that will actively help during those moments when you're feeling, well, less than your best.

And once you've figured out which tools work for you, you need to learn how best to employ them, and commit to utilising them whenever they're needed.

When learning, lean on the type of resources that work best for you as an individual, whether they're text-based, audio, visual or built on social interaction. It can also help when managing our lizard brain (which, going forward, I'll sometimes refer to as Mr Lizard) to cultivate an awareness of where we might sit on a scale of introversion/extroversion, and how this might vary according to our energy levels and environment.

Celebration

Appreciating natural tendencies

One of the books I read in the months following my return from Beijing was Susan Cain's enlightening *Quiet: The Power of Introverts in a World That Can't Stop Talking*. Having read it, I, for the first time, embraced my quietness. Rather than fighting against my natural tendencies, I wanted to celebrate them. I wanted the world to know I am not a naturally loud person, that I'd rather write than talk, and that I'm just as happy retreating into my own mind to rest as anywhere else.

Might your own disposition, beyond introversion or extroversion, be an issue or present opportunities for you? Maybe you're open-minded, imaginative, curious and willing to try new things. Do you seek excitement, novelty and thrills, often engaging in adventurous or risky activities? Perhaps you'd rather stick to what you know, the tried and tested, on safer ground. Some people tend to be agreeable, others more contrarian. Are you assertive, resilient, creative? Are you empathetic and able to understand and share the feelings of others, often showing compassion and support?

Developing self-awareness and appreciating natural tendencies are useful starting points when it comes to successfully managing the Lizard brain. Instead of beating myself up for being quiet in a group or in meetings, I accept my reluctance to speak unnecessarily. It's who I am, and I'm quite willing to write about it or whisper it from the rooftops.

Get It Right Next Time

Dealing with mistakes

Halting our Lizard in the middle of its fight, flight, freeze or fawn response to a frightening or stressful event, as it's happening, can feel nigh on impossible. But we do have control over Lizardy thinking (such as self-doubt and regret and other unhelpful reflection) in the minutes, hours and days after the event. This is particularly important to bear in mind if you've recently made a mistake, as rumination after the fact is both likely and harmful. We *can* avoid repeatedly replaying painful incidents in our mind.

The Lizard reacts. The human responds. Reactions are instinctive and immediate, and often based on fear and insecurities. They're often neither the most rational nor the most appropriate way to act. Responding, however, constitutes the rational behaviour and thoughts following an event. Responding means identifying what is happening or what has happened, understanding the situation and managing it with reason, compassion and co-operation.

Learn to override the Lizard and instead respond to mistakes with rational self-reflection that prioritises facts (e.g. I've made a mistake but it is fixable and I have got through far worse) over the fiction our Lizard tells us to protect us (e.g. this is a major catastrophe and everyone I know thinks worse of me). Most important of all, don't allow past reactions to dictate current behaviours. Don't allow them to become patterns.

Doing the work required to limit unhelpful reflection makes life easier and frees up mental energy for far more worthy pursuits. Guilt, self-doubt, regret and other emotions are temporary. But instead of dwelling on them, acknowledge them, allow them to exist and then dissolve in their own time. Feeling embarrassed when thinking back on mistakes is normal. No one is perfect, we all make them, and it helps when we take responsibility having done so. Not taking responsibility, or not doing our best to correct our error, is to make a second one.

We all make mistakes, and that's OK. They're a normal part of life.

The Man With the Red Face

Mistakes will happen (especially when the lizard brain handles things)

I'd picked up my daughter from school and we were driving home, heading up a two-lane hill near our house. As the traffic merged, another driver pulled alongside me. He was clearly trying to push in! Why couldn't he wait to get up the hill like me and everyone else in this lane? And why wasn't he even indicating to let me know he wanted to push in? And I bet he wouldn't even thank me after pushing his way in. My angry territorial instincts kicked in as this clown apparently tried to get in front of me. And – *get this!* – he was now talking to me through his half-down window! The audacity of the man.

I wound down my window and gave him an earful, something sweary about him not using his indicators, although I probably sounded more tabby than tiger.

As idiotic words tumbled from my mouth, I finally took a good look at the man and suddenly realised I'd made a big mistake. I stopped and turned to face my daughter.

"Er, this is actually a bit awkward," I said with a grimace.

"He's not trying to push in front of us. He's an old school mate I've known for 45 years. He's just trying to say hello. It's...

"That's it. I'm never going to live this down." My daughter winced.

That's an example of my amygdala, or lizard brain, taking over, having wrongly interpreted a normal event as a threat and getting involved aggressively before I could assess the situation rationally and behave like a grown-up.

My resident lizard had made me look completely stupid, again.

In another embarrassing incident, on a work trip, I repeatedly tried to get into my hotel room late one night with the office printer card. We've all done it. But not everyone immediately goes to reception and blames the hotel staff for giving them a faulty key card... My lizard brain was once again firmly in charge of my response. Moments later, after the staff had calmed me down with polite attention, they pointed out that an office printer card might not actually unlock a hotel room door. They showed me a key card, asked if I had a similar one, and I felt my face turn red before I scurried off upstairs and used mine to let myself into my room.

Crash

The Plimsoll line theory

Samuel Plimsoll MP campaigned in the 19th century for load lines – indicating the maximum depth to which a vessel could be safely immersed when loaded with cargo – to be painted on the side of ships to prevent them being overloaded and sinking in heavy weather or rough seas. (By that point, merchants transporting goods by sea already understood the importance of loading ships correctly and seafarers had been marking the sides of their vessels for hundreds of years, but still.) Some ships in the 19th century were so dangerous as a result of overloading and poor repair, they were known as 'coffin ships'.

Our heads are much like ships in this respect. When we're feeling overloaded with information, or in a challenging situation, or receiving lots of stimuli that require a response, our Plimsoll line is below the surface of the water and we feel rubbish. Then, when faced with a trigger – maybe a verbal nudge from a boss to work faster, or running into some kind of technology issue which trips us up, or perhaps a call from a bank asking difficult questions – we sink even lower.

I remember when I was in a sea of debt and had just returned from a family camping holiday in Cornwall. Already thinking about how I was going to pay the following month's bills having barely stepped through the front door, my kindly bank phoned me to ask about the £60 I'd spent in Homebase a couple of days earlier. They weren't particularly interested in the gazebo I'd had to buy to replace the broken one whose poles had been bent by strong winds one night, just before those same winds had launched it on to an unsuspecting camping party sleeping in the tent next door. They just wanted to know when I intended to clear my overdraft. I was more interested in how I was going to pay the mortgage, and whether I was soon going to be up on some tent-based assault charge.

Simply aiming for a much higher Plimsoll line at all times – in other words, a state of permanent happiness – so that there's no risk of feeling anxious when we are overloaded or triggered, is not the answer. That particular Promised Land doesn't exist.

Instead, aim to live "two notches above the Plimsoll line", to cultivate an "underlying sense of wellbeing and security", as brief therapist and life coach Alan Whitton suggests (brief therapy is short-term, solution-oriented therapy which focuses on setting and achieving goals, and targeting specific patterns rather than attempting to make broader personality changes). In other words, we need a buffer. This alternative approach leaves us more likely to keep our Plimsoll line where it should be: above water.

Striving for constant happiness – living 10 notches above the line – isn't sustainable. Aiming to live at '10' also means we have much further to fall when – not if – we're overloaded. When we're living unsustainably, hedonistically, and drama hits, a crash is inevitable and our line sinks below the water.

Part 3: science & scenarios

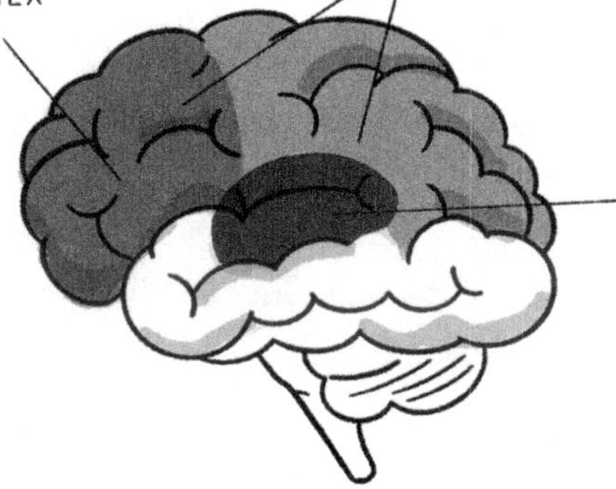

Human Behaviour

Why we do what we do

Consider this, from the website of charity Alzheimer's Research UK:

"The brain is the most complex thing in the universe. There are around 100 billion nerve cells (known as neurons) in the brain, each one connected to thousands of other cells.

"Your brain accounts for 2% of your bodyweight but uses about 20% of your energy. Brain cells use much more energy than other cells in your body and they're always active, even when you're asleep."

So why do we even have unhelpful negative thoughts if our brains are so clever and complex?

The prefrontal cortex (cortex derives from the Latin word for bark, as in the outer layer of trees) is the area of the brain associated with planning, decision-making, problem-solving and concentration: rational, 'human' responses. It enables us to consider complex issues and use reason to produce answers.

The amygdala, on the other hand, is among the oldest areas of the brain in human evolutionary terms and, because of this, is often referred to as the 'lizard brain' or 'reptilian brain'. It's a component of the brain's limbic system, where our fastest decisions are made, and "plays an important role in regulating emotions, especially the more 'negative' emotions, such as fear, aggression and anxiety"[1]. Everything we experience is processed in the limbic system first. It's where impulsiveness and instinct come from.

The midbrain sits at the top of the brainstem, between the prefrontal cortex and the amygdala, and helps us to apply meaning to our experiences.

The lizard brain developed first, followed by the midbrain, and, later, the prefrontal cortex. Our thought process follows the human brain's evolution: survival first, social relationships second, problem-solving last.

The amygdala's way of handling things goes back to a time when fear and aggression helped us survive in the wild. Our world has evolved but we're still wired to think prehistorically.

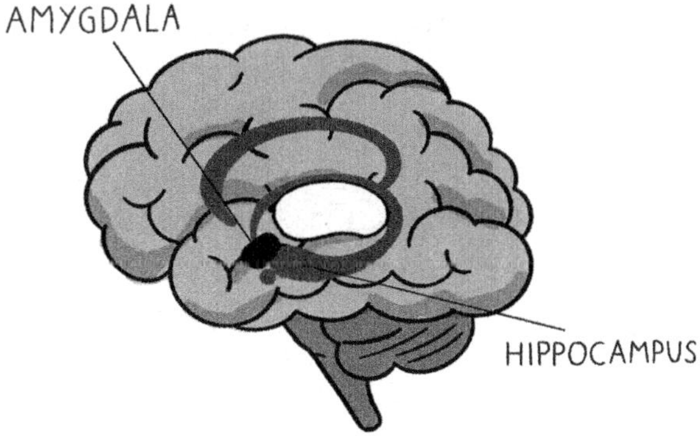

1 https://www.nhs.uk/mental-health/conditions/borderline-personality-disorder/causes/

Hanging Around

Mr Lizard is old

The amygdala, or lizard brain, can be your best friend or your worst enemy: it can save your life or it can get you into serious trouble.

The amygdala's name derives from the Greek word amygdale, meaning almond, because of its shape. It is one of the two major structures of the brain's limbic system, the other being the hippocampus, and is five times more powerful than our rational responses. Its reaction to triggers such as a perceived threat or meeting a potential mate can create an impossible-to-ignore feeling in our gut.

Mr Lizard's not leaving any time soon. Nor would you if you were that good at your job and boasted a glorious track record stretching back hundreds of thousands of years.

Unless stirred into action, instantaneously when necessary, Mr Lizard wants to either ignore information or spend as little time on it as possible. He's just hanging around, same as he's always done, waiting to do his thing. He sees the world as a battle to be won or lost.

Viva Las Vegas

The vagus nerve

The vagus nerve originates in the brainstem and is actually a pair of nerves. It's the longest cranial nerve in the body – which explains why it's named after the Latin word for wandering – and only mammals have it.

The vagus nerve is crucial in regulating our body's involuntary functions such as breathing, heart rate and the immune system and it does this by carrying messages between the brain and our internal organs, suggesting the inner organs are major sources of sensory information. This brain-organ connection is what gives us our 'gut feelings'.

The visceral excitement brought about by a new opportunity, our attraction to someone we've just met, or a sense of danger or that we're unwell can all generate gut feelings. They come from deep within us and form our intuition.

The vagus nerve's dorsal side forms the back and responds to signs of danger. The ventral side, the front of the vagus nerve, responds to safety cues, such as social engagement (receiving a smile or witnessing an act of kindness from a stranger, for example), deep breathing or mindful thinking. Both sides may be activated when we're trying to determine whether situations or people are safe, dangerous or life-threatening.

The vagus nerve is part of the parasympathetic nervous system, which governs the 'rest and digest' processes and relaxes the body after periods of stress or danger. In those moments of pressure, our sympathetic fight-or-flight responses are activated, and processes that are less important in emergencies or times of stress, such as digestion, are slowed.

The question is: can we consciously affect our vagus state? That is, can we decide to move our bodies from a state of stress to a state of relaxation? Can we counteract our natural fight-or-flight response in order to feel calmer, clearer, more compassionate, more connected? Yes, but more on that later.

Strangers

Trusting your gut

Our lizard brain – our intuition, our gut – is exceptionally good at keeping us alive. It often gets a read on someone before we're even consciously aware of that impression. As entrepreneur, podcaster and *Dragon's Den* investor Steven Bartlett shared on social media: "Your gut can spot ego, character flaws and negative intentions because your gut instinct doesn't overlook past lessons like your mind does. You have to trust your gut when it comes to choosing the people you surround yourself with."

Thousands of years ago, we might have spotted a hungry tiger coming towards us rather than a speeding bus, and then Lizard would've prepared us to deal with the perceived danger instantaneously by urging us to run away or hide. Fighting a hungry tiger would presumably have been the wrong move.

While the threat of hungry predators may have abated, we might have to deal with negative comments on social media, critical emails from a client or boss, or anxiety triggered by an upcoming event we must attend but would rather not. A perceived threat triggers our fight-or-flight state.

Sometimes our intuition shouts. Other times it whispers. I was on a train with my younger daughter in 2022, one stop from home, when I heard my intuition come through, loud and clear, as I considered whether I should offer to help the stranger a few seats away.

His face was spattered with blood, his knuckles were red-raw and his bike looked even more beaten up than he did. I thought briefly. I didn't have long before we reached our stop.

Had he been knocked off his bike, scraped his knuckles on the road and survived? Maybe he was a painter and decorator and had got a bit clumsy with the red paint. I wanted to know his story. I wanted to make sure he was OK. Should I go over? Hmm.

As I pondered, I knew – I could *feel* – I was wasting my time. While I was deliberating, I'd felt my intuition ring out like a bell and I had full trust in that feeling: leave well alone. Something wasn't right about that person or his situation. Maybe it was his vacant thousand-yard stare. Maybe he'd cycled to his victim's house, attacked him and taken a hiding for his trouble. What if he'd got frustrated with a non-indicating motorist and got into a fight? Maybe he'd had a scrap with a hungry tiger.

If I approached the man and he lashed out, it'd be my own stupid fault, so I left him to it, telling myself we just can't help everyone who might need it. Offering assistance in that moment felt wrong.

Just Can't Get Enough

Dopamine and other neurotransmitters

Serotonin, oxytocin and endorphins all act as hormones and, as well as dopamine, produce our positive emotions. They are neurotransmitters produced in the brainstem, and we need each one to feel emotionally balanced. We're able to produce endorphins and dopamine on our own. To produce serotonin and oxytocin, however, we need other people.

Serotonin influences our appetite, behaviour and thinking. It improves sleep, stabilises mood and strengthens human bonds, such as those between parent and child, coach and player, leader and team. It imbues us with feelings of confidence, pride, status and respect.

Oxytocin encourages us to serve others. When we help someone else, we feel good for helping, and they feel good because they've benefited from whatever it was we did for them. It's a win-win. It's oxytocin at work. Donating money or time, sending a birthday card, hugging, high-fiving, holding hands, petting your dog or cat and cooking for loved ones will all stimulate oxytocin production.

Endorphins are the body's natural painkillers, released to relieve pain or stress, and create a general feeling of wellbeing. Their name comes from the term endogenous morphine: endogenous means 'produced by an organism' (in this case, our bodies), and morphine refers to the opioid painkiller whose actions they mimic. There are about 20 types of endorphin, including the particularly powerful and much studied beta-endorphin, which is associated with a 'runner's high'.

A great friend of mine, Jon, regularly competes in Ironman triathlons. They involve swimming 2.4 miles (3.8km), cycling the equivalent of London to Loughborough (112 miles/180km) and then running a marathon in what's widely regarded as one of the world's toughest one-day sporting events.

"After turbo training on a Saturday," Jon told me of his riding on a static bike indoors, "from 6am until midday, the boost lasts until Tuesday. Training makes me feel almost indestructible."

We also release endorphins when we laugh, fall in love, have sex and eat a delicious meal.

And finally, dopamine. Dopamine influences memory, mood, sleep, learning, concentration and body movements. It's also highly addictive and for that reason is potentially dangerous. It enables us to feel pleasure, satisfaction and motivation. When we feel good having achieved a goal, reached a target or won some money, it's because we feel a surge of dopamine.

Dopamine can be released when we consume nicotine, exercise, win a game or contest, earn money, engage in criminal activity, sex, driving, gambling or social media. Alcohol and many illegal drugs cause a surge of dopamine too, which is partly why people become addicted to them. Some people are addicted to the dopamine hit they get when they experience anger, fear (from participating in extreme sports, driving fast, watching horror films or riding huge rollercoasters, for example), violence (groups of rival football fans fighting) or intimidation, either as a bully or perhaps as the bullied, such as when, for example, someone inadvertently becomes addicted to the drama and fear abusive partners bring into their lives.

Some people don't stay in abusive relationships just because they're scared to leave or feel trapped by their circumstances. Research such as that published in the Journal of Social and Personal Relationships shows that many develop a deep emotional attachment to their abuser through a phenomenon known as 'traumatic bonding'. It's a cycle: abuse, then kindness, then more abuse. The brain clings to the moments of affection, making it incredibly hard to walk away. The push and pull become addictive, creating a dependency not just on the person but on the drama itself: the highs, the lows, the constant emotional turmoil.

On social media, we're hooked on the prospect of a new, potentially positive, outcome: just like fruit machines when you put your money in and press the button, your brain can't wait to see what turns up.

Why would part of our own brain encourage us to use or engage in things that offer little or no discernible benefit to us just to get a hit?

It's how we're wired.

Dopamine makes us feel good when we engage in activities that keep the species alive, such as eating, and then it gets abused when we want more of whatever it is we enjoy intensely, and are able to very easily access it.

Another reason social media, some online games, junk food and takeaways are so addictive is because they're deliberately designed and manufactured to be so. So, for instance, on top of the hit you'd get anyway from eating junk food because of the high sugar and salt content, all sorts of chemicals and ingredients – such as high-fructose corn syrup and monosodium glutamate – are added to food to make it even tastier and keep us coming back for more.

Dopamine can be destructive if the amount in our body is out of whack. Having low levels can reduce motivation and focus, and increase procrastination. Too much dopamine in some parts of the brain and not enough in others is linked to being more competitive, aggressive and having poor impulse control.

Safe From Harm

Our stress hormone

Cortisol is a neurotransmitter which helps to protect us from danger. Its release is the first stage of our fight-or-flight response. When cortisol is released, systems which aren't necessary for survival are shut down. Oxytocin levels dip and adrenaline flows, giving us the energy needed to fight or run away. Cortisol leaves our bloodstream as soon as the threat has passed. But sometimes, our brains get it wrong, and release cortisol when there isn't any real danger, resulting in constant feelings of fear or paranoia.

I used to have a problem with sneezing in the office. I'd feel a sneeze coming, and it'd be accompanied by a sense of danger and panic that the resulting noise would draw attention which would lead to me being 'found out' and then slung out for incompetence. I (my rational brain) knew it was nonsense but I still believed the story.

The sneeze would roll along and I'd try to stop it, as I took the advice of my unconscious brain, the Lizard within. He'd suggest I stifle the sneeze so I could carry on hiding and stay 'safe'. He didn't want to be noticed, rejected or become a burden, so I felt danger when there was none. In fact, trying to stifle sneezes made matters worse: they would force themselves out regardless. Trying to keep a lid on the natural noise meant it found its way out from a corner of my mouth and sounded like I was letting the air out of a balloon for comic effect. And of course, that would grab everyone's attention.

By using some of the methods I explain later, I managed to navigate this issue. I was able to sit at my desk, sneeze when I needed to – like most people – and not get thrown out or even asked what I was doing there.

Every Time A Bell Rings

Types of Lizard

Let's meet Mr Lizard. While everybody has a Lizard, not all Lizards are the same. Mine, for example, will stir into action immediately only when he really needs to. Occasionally, however, he'll take his time waking up, then assess the situation as he stretches and makes himself a cup of tea before lighting a cigarette and only then offering a response.

Other people's Lizards, on the other hand, do things very differently. Theirs are always on shift, ready to leap into action immediately, fists at the ready, every time their phone rings, they hear a knock at the door or a baby crying. Every time, in fact, there's the slightest hint of a threat they believe needs dealing with.

Some Lizards would rather lie and deny, blame and complain, than take responsibility. Such tendencies can leave the person whose Lizard does this feeling confused, guilty or defensive if this lack of responsibility is picked up on by those around them and condemned. Other Lizards retain a focus on truth and justice, which can leave their owner feeling frustrated if an incident or something someone has said needs picking up on and calling out – at least in their Lizard's view – but is difficult to do so for some reason. Similarly, the things that get my dopamine flowing might not necessarily light you up in the same way. And what you love to do might not be your best friend's idea of fun. Her Lizard might be wild compared with yours, causing your friend all sorts of mischief.

Lizard really knows what he wants. He knows exactly how to get it, when to jump in and take complete control, instantaneously, of your thinking. And he knows when to rescue you before you've even had time to realise what's going on. He's that quick. Before you assessed the situation, having stepped into the road without looking properly – perhaps because the friend you were with at the time wrongly said it was safe to do so – he saved you. You might be shaking and in shock, but you realise you're alive, and that's thanks to Lizard. He's selfish. He doesn't want to perish under a bus. He keeps you safe to keep himself safe.

Lizard knows when and how to convince you (so easily) to do something naughty because you (he) will enjoy it even if you (the real you this time, the rational you) might have to later fix the consequences of that thing because it wasn't in your best interests or of those around you.

Lizard is present when we're browsing and in buying mode. In fact, he'll often actually decide what gets bought. We buy and decide with emotion, then justify with logic. For example, someone might buy a pair of shoes they don't need because they couldn't resist, having allowed emotion to get the better of them. They later seek to justify their decision by reasoning, "I had to get them because they were on special offer, and they were the only pair in the shop."

Or maybe their head was telling them one thing – "I should leave the pub in the next five minutes or it'll be more expensive to get home and I might upset my partner" – but their Lizard was in the driving seat and deciding for them, leaving the rational brain to explain later: "Yes, I missed my train home but I had to stay for those extra beers because so-and-so turned up and I hadn't seen them in ages."

So our Lizards aren't going anywhere, we can't be 'cured' of them, nor can we change thoughts and behaviours we're neither aware of nor able to make sense of. We must therefore aim to do three important things:

1. Spot the behavioural patterns provoked by our Lizard.

2. Understand why those patterns occur: might we be repeating what we were exposed to as we grew up? For example, Dad deals with stress by drinking, and as we get stressed we find ourselves drinking too. Step-dad was controlling, and we find ourselves attracted to someone who turns out to be controlling. Unhealthy behaviours often serve as coping mechanisms for underlying psychological issues such as stress, anxiety, depression, or low self-esteem. People may engage in these behaviours as a way to alleviate emotional discomfort temporarily. Despite the negative consequences, an individual (or their Lizard) may perceive some benefits from their unhealthy behaviours, such as temporary relief from discomfort or social acceptance within certain circles. These perceived benefits can outweigh the drawbacks in the individual's mind, making it difficult to change. Our environment might also

give us contributing factors – peer pressure, family dynamics and workplace culture among them – for repeating unhealthy behaviour.

Books including Eckhart Tolle's *The Power of Now*, *Mindset: The New Psychology of Success* by Carol Dweck, and *Change Your Thinking Change Your Life* by Brian Tracy helped me to gain more self-awareness, and I recommend all of them.

3. Finally, we must manage the patterns to develop a more flexible and resilient mindset and try to consciously prevent our Lizard from holding us back. Behaviours can become ingrained habits that are difficult to break. We might recognise our own unhealthy behaviour but breaking the habit requires conscious effort and often support from others. The strategies I explain in Part 4 are designed to help manage negative patterns of behaviour, build resilience and achieve more peace of mind.

Stir It Up

Know when your Lizard is likely to stir

What stirs our Lizards into action? Well, that depends on all sorts of factors – our environment, how energised we're feeling (or not), the pressure we're under, for example – and the type of Lizard we're talking about (see p.63). Of course there are states common to us all when we can assume that everyone's Lizard is awake and ready for action, such as when we're scared or feeling anxious, but what is it specifically that triggers those feelings of fear or anxiety in the first place?

We clearly can't prevent our Lizard leaping into action when he spots or senses danger way before our rational brain does, and we wouldn't want to even if we could, but it's worth developing an awareness of the anxiety-inducing situations (triggers you may have developed in childhood as a result of your upbringing) that are likely to arouse him.

How do you deal with stress through overworking, for example, or when you know you have an exam approaching, or when you have to present to a group? What do your body and brain do when you're in a large crowd or when plans fall apart? Your Lizard might perceive a certain person or group of people or a particular place where you've felt pain in the past, or a certain time of year – Christmas or an anniversary, for example – as particularly threatening. Or he might be aroused when faced with the unknown or temptation.

Examples of when a Lizard might be stirred into action:

- When outside his comfort zone
- When feeling like an impostor
- When pleasure or success exceed familiar levels
- When he's tired
- When it's late
- When facing a familiar fear
- In the company of a group
- When the goalposts move: for example, when instructions from a boss, client or a figure of authority change with little or no notice
- When another driver acts without respect, consideration or gratitude

If we're more aware of when those conditions that trigger fear and panic materialise, we become more capable of managing our lizard brain satisfactorily. Aim to shift from unconscious default behaviours, thoughts and biological responses by noticing, becoming aware, taking control, and making different decisions. This could mean visualising the pressure you expect to feel at a particular time or in a certain situation and working on replacing negative thoughts with positive ones (perhaps by writing positive words in discreet but helpful places to give you a boost just when you need it). The coach of former tennis player Johanna Konta encouraged her to use visualisation techniques and instilled trigger words such as "keep fighting" and "you can do it" into her mind to keep her at ease during high-pressure moments on court.

Visualising not just the outcome you desire but focusing on smaller achievements could also be helpful. In practical terms, maybe taking control and taking steps to increase your chances of success involves practising a presentation until you know it off by heart, establishing a manageable revision schedule which you do with a friend and then quiz each other in order to hold each other accountable, or working through a set of breathing exercises before an exam.

Under The Bridge

Moving beyond comfort zones

"Are you willing to be uncomfortable for five minutes?
Exercising is easier once you've started the workout.
Conversation is easier once you're already talking.
Writing is easier once you're in the middle of it.
Many rewards in life will elude you if you're not
willing to be a little uncomfortable at first."

– James Clear, author of the *New York Times* bestseller, *Atomic Habits*

Our lizard brain's discomfort is temporary and often brief when we find ourselves in, or are preparing for, an anxiety-inducing situation, but that won't necessarily lessen our apprehension or the unease we feel as a result of his perceptions.

Meeting new people, starting at a new school, college or university, or a new job, facing a challenging domestic situation – all can trigger significant discomfort. The unfamiliar can be very stressful because it's full of what our lizard brain perceives as threats or dangers...until it susses them out and realises there are no actual threats or dangers and the unfamiliar becomes the familiar. What is it that gets Lizard up, dressed and ready for battle before you've even had time to put the kettle on? Where does he hang out? Under the bridge, perhaps...

I'm reminded of the Norwegian fairytale, *Three Billy Goats Gruff*: three billy goats are getting hungry because there's almost no grass left for them to eat near where they live so they must cross a river to reach the beautiful, lush meadow on the other side.

The bridge is near the goats' house (more of a bungalow really – everybody knows goats don't live in houses). And under that bridge lives a nasty, hungry troll who'd love to eat the goats or anyone else hoping to pop round and cross the river. Terrible host, this troll.

The smallest goat crosses first. He gets stopped by the troll who threatens to eat him. But Little Goat convinces Troll not to eat him because his brother, the next goat to cross, has put on a few pounds recently and will therefore provide a nicer meal. Troll says OK, fair enough, and lets Little Goat cross unscathed. Happy Little Goat. Next up, Middle-size Goat. Same thing happens: troll wants to eat goat, goat convinces troll to wait for larger brother. Goat crosses bridge unharmed. Third goat – Big Goat – gets on the bridge. Troll has a word, trying to convince Big Goat he's toast. But Big Goat won't have it, challenges Troll and dares him to eat him. Troll has a pop, Big Goat swings an uppercut and knocks Troll off the bridge and into the river. Troll's gone (terrible swimmer as well as a poor host), and Big Goat joins his brothers in the field of dreams where they all eat happily ever after.

Sometimes the battle is in getting yourself through the Great Unknown to find out what's on the other side. As Friedrich Nietzsche wrote: "No one can construct for you the bridge upon which precisely you must cross the stream of life, no one but you yourself alone."

Growth happens when we leave our comfort zones. You can always go back but it's important to leave the house every now and then, get uncomfortable, and learn to love that as-yet uncharted territory.

What A Waste

Wasting time on impostor syndrome

"Boris Johnson is probably the archduke of not having impostor syndrome. You don't lead the country in a two-year-long, ego-driven, blindfolded cancan through a minefield, stopping only to machinegun the British public's money directly at your very best friends before going back to a flat those same friends paid to decorate to celebrate the fact you can carry on your bloated, masturbatory Winston Churchill fantasy, at everybody's expense, until the country is literally drained dry. You have to be dragged out by your ankles leaving your fingernails embedded in the doorframe... Do you think that man wasted a second on self-examination?" – Troy Hawke

That's a good question and, thankfully, I am not Boris Johnson. A consequence of not being Boris Johnson however is that I have spent more than a few seconds on self-examination, overthinking and impostor syndrome.

Tendencies to doubt our place at a particular desk or in a particular office or as part of a better team, to feel we somehow don't deserve to be there, are stifling. They can appear in the workplace, in a sporting environment, in social settings. While it might at times feel like this specific flavour of self-doubt is a ridiculous waste of time, there is some benefit to this kind of self-examination, for some people at least: sometimes we aren't up to the job. We shouldn't ignore our intuition when it's telling us we might be better suited doing something different. I wonder how the UK might have benefited had Boris Johnson and his ilk listened to that tiny niggling voice on the blue moons it whispers that running the country may not have been his forte.

"That person next to you?" Here we go, Lizard's piping up. "Compare him and his career with yours. Ha ha ha, good one. Remind me again why you're here..."

Overthinking is generally a wasteful pursuit. As Steven Bartlett says, overthinking "prevents progress and kills happiness. But no amount of anxiety," he adds, "will change your future and no amount of regret can change your past. The key is acceptance. Accepting imperfection, accepting uncertainty and accepting that some things are beyond your control."

Sabotage

Turning good things bad

Sometimes, when things are good or we're having a nice time, our Lizard will turn those things or occasions sour. For example, a couple have enjoyed a great day out but before they know it, they're in the middle of an argument that one of them started.

This is because Lizards prefer the familiar. He might not like familiar people, surroundings, events or so on but when he understands them, he knows where any real or potential threats might come from. He feels as though he's on safe ground. However, he regards the unfamiliar – and that can include happiness – as being fraught with danger, real or potential. Rather than be caught out, he'll disrupt.

Therefore, our Lizard might cause us to sabotage a pleasant experience or relationship simply because he doesn't know where it might lead, even if that is your happiness.

Psychologist Gay Hendricks calls such issues "upper limit problems" in his book *The Big Leap*. "Each of us," he wrote, "has an inner thermostat setting that determines how much love, success and creativity we allow ourselves to enjoy. When we exceed our inner thermostat setting, we will often do something to sabotage ourselves, causing us to drop back into the old familiar zone where we feel secure."

Sometimes then, in order to achieve greater happiness, we must identify, understand and manage those occasions when our Lizard is getting in the way. It might be when we come into a bit of money and allow it to slip through our fingers as quickly as it arrived, or it could be when we reach a certain point early in a new relationship and find ourselves fabricating reasons why we need to split up. Lizard's fear of the unknown is at the heart of his intervention.

I'm So Tired

Lizards target the tired

"One of the most productive things we can do is rest."

– Arsène Wenger

Psychotherapist Owen O'Kane understands the importance of rest. "You've got to really learn how to look after yourself. You've got to be able to recognise when you begin to tire, when you start to feel symptoms of burning out. You need to be able to recognise when that's happening.

"Where do you take the gaps in your day? What are you doing to take care of yourself? Who are the people you're surrounding yourself with?"

At sporting events, work days are usually long and intense. The workload doesn't always make it easy to take breaks, and I happily accept this as part of the job. And I understand that when I'm tired my lizard brain might try to creep in and hijack my thinking. My Lizard loves it when I'm tired. It's as if the rational me has opened the front door of my house just before I take a nap in front of the telly. My eyes face the TV but, before they're even closed, Lizard has quietly crept into the house and is now in the same room as me.

When I'm tired and in company, I tend to go quiet. Sparkling wit and engaging conversation are the first things to go.

Here's an example:

I'm in a pleasant restaurant with good company. The conversation is light, funny and sharp. It's fast-paced. But the warmth of the room combined with my early start to meet my deadlines has made me feel oh so tired. I can barely keep up. Inside my head, I don't notice as my Lizard slides into his favourite armchair in the corner on the other side of the room. He kicks off his shoes and lights a cigar. He sits back, puffing, grinning, waiting. Very soon, he'll be in charge of my thinking, and he knows it.

Friends at events have seen me bend my run, to use a football term, to unexpectedly swerve a sociable dinner at the last minute and avoid this very situation. Nothing personal, just tiredness.

In the restaurant, I've been quiet for a couple of minutes now. And if I've noticed, my friends must have too. In my head, my silence feels more like 10 or 20 minutes and is feeling increasingly awkward and uncomfortable.

"You're quiet," Lizard says menacingly, partially obscured behind a plume of cigar smoke. I can see just enough to notice his grin has gone.

"Everything alright?" he asks, the smoke fading. I'm not at all engaged in the friendly conversation going on around me. I feel hungry. My quietness is making me feel anxious. I could sleep right now.

"Pardon?"

"I said, 'You're quiet.' Everything alright?"

My Lizard knows everything is not alright. He's spotted my vulnerability and made it worse.

"Have you had a good trip, Paul? What's been your highlight?" A photographer friend sitting opposite me is being friendly and I struggle to reply. He might as well have asked me what I did on my 15th birthday. My lips are sealed and the photographer is suddenly distracted and absorbed by something funny and clearly more interesting going on at the other end of the table.

But I'm slightly more energised after sipping a glass of wine and eating some bread.

I feel better still after finishing a bowl of pasta. I make a joke, people laugh, and Lizard is asleep in the armchair, extinguished cigar clinging to his lip.

Sometimes the gulf between agonising discomfort and feeling part of the group can feel enormous. Most of the time, it's only a meal, a nap, a shared moment or a smile away.

After Midnight

Lizards love the small hours

You're in bed. It's 02:44 and you can't sleep. Your mind's racing. You're turning over a few things in your head and it's not going well. Actually, you are asleep – the 'real' you, that is. But your Lizard? He's wide awake, running amok and running the show, full of unhelpful reflection and predictions. You started off feeling bad, now you feel worse. Into a torrent flows a torrent.

Tip: don't listen to your Lizard after midnight. He will not help you rest. He knows you can't resist his nonsense in the small hours, which is why you're prone to overthinking and catastrophising, and turning events – real or imagined – over and over in your head when you should be asleep. If this is you, thank your Lizard for his input, then ignore everything he says until the rational you wakes up in the morning.

Getting enough good quality sleep is essential for sound mental health, and the chances of that happening increase exponentially when you ignore your late-night Lizard.

Scared

Fear is normal

David Bowie avoided **flying** between autumn 1972 and spring 1977. A premonition in which he died in a plane crash was reportedly enough to keep him out of the sky and travelling by boat, bus and train as he toured.

In a 2014 interview on his recovery from addiction, Metallica's James Hetfield said: **"I've been afraid of responsibility my whole life, not wanting to take responsibility for myself."**

When asked in 2021 what his greatest fear was, Dave Grohl said, **"Being stuck in an elevator. I'm not a claustrophobic type but for whatever reason there's something about being stuck in an elevator."**

Ozzy Osbourne said in 2018: **"I tell you what I am scared of – rats. They've got so many diseases we don't have the cure for."** Freddie Mercury was terrified of **spiders**. The 2018 Olympic downhill champion Sofia Goggia, meanwhile, is petrified of **snakes**.

When you're scared, your Lizard is on high alert for anything that might make a bad situation worse, anything that validates the story he's already telling you that there are things to be afraid of all around you.

But when we face fear head-on, it diminishes. Its power decreases. Between January 2018 and September 2019, the psychologist Dr Pippa Grange taught the England men's football team to face and decrease their fears by encouraging the players to be more open, to share personal stories and to shed inhibitions. This input, placed among a larger package of winning behaviours, helped those players in 2018 to reach the World Cup semi-finals for the first time in 28 years and, in 2020, to compete in their first European Championship final.

Our Lips Are Sealed

What will they think?

There's a question that often gets in the way of us achieving everything we're capable of, and Mr Lizard is more than happy to oblige in asking it: what will they think?

If I aim for a lofty ambition, what will they think?

If I apply for that job I think I'd be great at, what will they think?

If I attempt to speak in a foreign language when abroad with colleagues, what will they think?

In a 1995 academic paper, social psychologist Roy Baumeister and professor of psychology and neuroscience Mark Leary argued that humans are naturally inclined to establish and sustain a sense of belonging. "[We are]…driven by the need to belong...likewise, people prefer achievements that are validated, recognized and valued by other people over solitary achievement." In other words, we care what our friends, family, teammates or colleagues think because those people are our tribe, our group.

We need to feel a bond with them for two reasons. First, in ancient times we relied on our tribe to survive: we could sleep when protected by others; we could eat food gathered by them. Second, we need to feel fulfilled, and that often comes when we've contributed in a meaningful way to the group. We like the hit of serotonin and oxytocin.

Sometimes we worry our contribution won't be seen as positive. We're concerned we'll let down the group in some way, leaving us feeling unfulfilled, shunned and in danger, or looking foolish.

Our lizard steps in to keep us 'safe'. Maybe I'll stop chasing that goal. Perhaps I'll ask my question in English instead of trying to articulate it in a foreign language – or perhaps I'll remain silent. I don't want them to think less of me. Sometimes life's easier when we avoid having to justify our decisions to the group.

If we can resist the lizard voice in our heads that makes us afraid of judgement and failure, we can achieve so much more, and expand our comfort zones too.

PART 4: the strategies

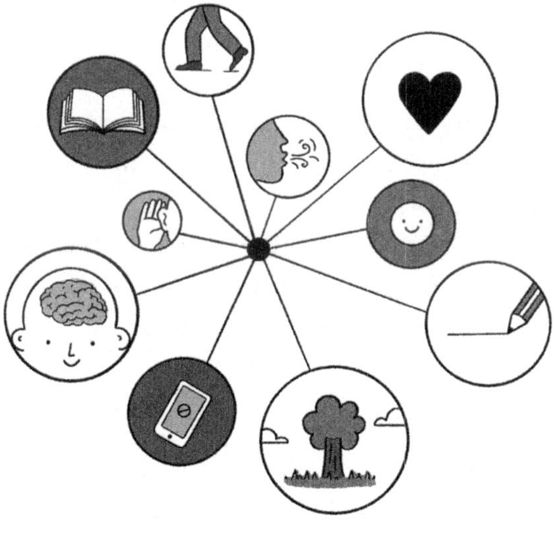

Over and Over

Repetition is key

"We are what we repeatedly do. Excellence, then, is not an act, but a habit."

– Will Durant, historian and philosopher

Speaking to the physician, author and broadcaster Rangan Chatterjee on his BBC radio programme *Out of Hours* in February 2022, psychologist Dr Julie Smith explained, "Wellness isn't boxes. We're not either 'well' or 'unwell'. We're all on this kind of spectrum and we move up and down it. Your physical health can deteriorate but you might not consider yourself [...] 'unwell'. And it's the same with mental health.

"We can have those normal fluctuations, and there are things we can do to help that, to boost our mental wellness in the same way we do for our physical health.

"There are certain lifestyle choices and things that we would do to boost our physical health and I think we have to start seeing mental health in that way because lots of people feel they're at the mercy of how they feel, or at the mercy of their mood or emotional state, and they're not really as educated as [they] could be around what [they] can do to help [them] selves."

So our physical and mental health fluctuate. This is normal. By that same token, our happiness levels also fluctuate. Generally speaking, we're neither merely 'happy' nor 'unhappy'. This, too, is normal and healthy. Consequently, it's not realistic to aim for happiness all the time.

Dr Smith reiterates that we should prepare for the perfectly normal times when we're feeling less than happy. Those periods when life is tough or not going our way can feel like they're dragging on for ever. Those are the times when Lizard is more likely to voice an opinion or offer a skewed perspective that might not serve our best interests.

When our mental health is poor, we can try to improve it by taking more exercise, drinking less alcohol, sleeping more, eating healthily, using medicine or seeking professional medical help. We can also actively choose not to listen to negative or unhelpful thoughts, get outdoors, list reasons to be grateful or deploy mindfulness or breathing techniques.

Problems are exacerbated when we ignore them, when we try to block them out with drink, drugs, food or sex, or when we want to tackle them but are unsure how or where or when to get help. At such times, we might just leave them and hope they fix themselves. Or perhaps we don't even notice we've got a problem in the first place.

Practising mental wellness techniques during smooth periods makes them easier to use when required.

"It's really tough to begin using these skills when things are already really, really bad," Dr Smith continued. "It's much easier to practise a skill when things are OK, so [you can use it] when you need it. The idea is to get practising ways to look after yourself when you're not in desperate need of it."

Kevin Sinfield is a rugby union coach having played rugby league as the captain of Leeds Rhinos. Many fans of the sport believe he was one of the best kickers in the game's history. He made over 500 appearances for Leeds and was part of seven Rhinos Super League title-winning teams.

He's also completed seven marathons in seven days, seven ultramarathons in seven days and run from Leicester to Leeds to raise money in support of his friend and former teammate Rob Burrow, who at the time of writing is suffering with motor neurone disease.

On his approach to kicking for points during important matches, Sinfield told Adrian Chiles in a BBC radio interview:

"I trusted in my prep. I trusted in the fact that I'd spent hours and hours on the training field kicking. You only become concerned or stressed or worried about something when you've not done your homework, or you've not done enough practice, and I knew I'd done that."

For those big moments during important matches, Sinfield had prepared as well as he could have by doing the same thing over and over again.

This prep meant he was able to "flick into autopilot" when there was an important kick coming up. "If there was a big kick to be taken – or any kick, for that matter – I'd very quickly flick over from the rugby player to the goal kicker and perform my job, my skill, the best I could, and straight afterwards flick straight back into the rugby player."

Our lizard brain and our rational brain don't work separately. They work differently. They try to work together, but they can and do clash, and because the lizard brain is more powerful and more primitive, it often wins the struggle to dominate our thinking. One of the best ways then to perform at your best during moments of intense pressure, and manage that inner struggle, is to put the work in and practise beforehand. Then you can trust in that work and shut down the Lizard when it matters most.

Strategy 1: Complete Control

Place your confidence with care

Confidence, for many people, is a by-product of their ability to succeed in past endeavours.

These endeavours, such as winning a race, getting elected or passing an exam, are outcomes and while we can sometimes improve our chances of success in our endeavours through practice, as in Kevin Sinfield's story on p.88, outcomes are often beyond our control. Therefore, deriving confidence from successful outcomes is a flawed strategy, which can lead to either too much confidence or not enough. It's a lizardy way of thinking.

The alternative is more rational: basing your confidence on doing your best, over which you have complete control, rather than an outcome over which you have none or very little. Do your best and learn to be OK with the consequences, no matter what they are, safe in the knowledge that you did all you could.

Dr Steve Peters is a clinical psychiatrist who's worked with Liverpool FC, the England football team, seven-time world snooker champion Ronnie O'Sullivan, and the Olympic cycling gold medallists Sir Chris Hoy and Victoria Pendleton. He's also the author of *The Chimp Paradox*, in which he uses the analogy of a chimp where others use a crocodile or a lizard. He wrote:

"With this choice we can see that the normal state for the Human is confidence because you can always do your best and deal with consequences, and therefore there is no fear. Whereas the normal state for the Chimp is variable confidence, with a lot of fear, based around consequences and possible failure."

Strategy 2: Don't Be So Hard On Yourself

Forgive yourself – no one's perfect

Pay attention to the language you use to describe yourself and talk to yourself. If your lizard brain always reaches for unhelpful language to describe you or something involving you, pause and remember: you do not have to accept as fact what you're saying about yourself to other people and inside your head. You don't have to settle for that negative self-talk. In fact, if you always view yourself negatively, it's incredibly *important* that you don't settle for that.

What are your core beliefs about yourself? What were you always told? What psychological blueprint was drawn up as you were growing up? Such messages – for example, 'You're not very bright. You won't do well at school' – become internalised to the extent that we carry them into adulthood.

If your internal voice uses language you wouldn't use when talking to a friend or stranger, choose nicer things to think and say about yourself. Be your own internal coach, not a negative commentator. That's a simple and effective starting point.

It's worth noting here the American journalist and author Maria Shriver, who wrote:

"Self-empathy is the acknowledgment that, like all human beings, you deserve understanding and compassion. To truly practise self-empathy to its fullest, you must be willing to use it even when you trip over your own feet and make mistakes that leave you feeling embarrassed or wishing you had stayed home."

Dr Steve Peters was asked in a radio interview for one tip he could offer listeners, a strategy he'd used himself for greater mental resilience. He replied: "To be more forgiving of myself."

The next time you're self-critical, ask yourself: where's the evidence suggesting that that criticism is true? Where's the justification? Find the positive 'what ifs' – for example, 'What if I ignore my self-criticism and *do* apply for that job, and I get an interview? I can talk to people, listen well and show them I'm keen….' Or, 'What if I apply for my dream university? I *am* clever enough and I might actually get in – and if I don't, at least I will have tried and gained experience, and there are other universities which are also very good.'

Acknowledge that you too deserve to be happy and can be ambitious. Give yourself permission to try to achieve good things. How would you feel if, after deciding to choose nicer words to think and say about yourself, you achieved success? Forgive. Be kind to yourself.

Strategy 3: Say Hello, Wave Goodbye

Acknowledge, evaluate, decide, act

In difficult moments, remember this: you don't have to accept your lizard brain's perspective. Some of its suggestions – to fight, run away or freeze – in response to deep-rooted irrational fears, aren't helpful. You can say thanks for the perspective but it's not for me because it's not grounded in reality.

To make room for better, you have to know what 'better' is, or at least know what you're not willing to accept. Acknowledge, evaluate, decide, act: say hello to the Lizard, then wave goodbye?

Possibly.

For example, as I write this book, I know there's even harder work to come later when I begin to promote the product to get it in front of potential readers, people who might not know me.

I always find marketing my books to be a barrier because self-promotion doesn't come naturally to me. But I also know that without marketing, my book – with all the work, time and financial investment I've put into it – will not reach the number of people I want it to.

So what holds me back?

Fear, and what Steven Pressfield calls Resistance.

Pressfield is an American author who wrote for 27 years before he got his first novel published. During that time, he worked 21 different jobs in eleven states, including as an advertising copywriter, a schoolteacher, barman, fruit-picker and a Hollywood screenwriter.

He has written extensively, particularly in his bestselling book *The War of Art,* on Resistance – "fear, self-doubt, procrastination, perfectionism, all the forms of self-sabotage that stop us from doing our work and realising our dreams". I need to listen to him for frequent reminders that Resistance, which is essentially lizard-based thinking, can be managed successfully. If he can do it, so can I. I can get out of my own way.

Having been guilty of allowing my lizard brain to keep me 'safe' by keeping me invisible, away from social media and pretty much all other forms of marketing, I now better understand this force that can slow our progress or stop us striving for achievement.

What will I do about it? What *can* I do about it? I can detach from it.

Detaching from negative thoughts and feelings is an idea I learned in two books: *Think Like a Monk,* by Jay Shetty, and Dr Julie Smith's *Why Has Nobody Told Me This Before?*. Acceptance of thoughts and feelings is optional. We can detach ourselves from them. Stick to the facts. Thoughts and feelings are not facts. Separated and evaluated, they each amount to merely one possible perspective, and the lizard brain is heavily involved in generating it.

First, acknowledge each thought and every feeling you're experiencing. Express, privately if you prefer, the feeling you're experiencing. Instead of simply turning thoughts and feelings over and over in your head, giving them power, strength and a permanent invite to your internal dialogue, press pause in your mind. Try Owen O'Kane's 'helicopter method': first, lift your mind's eye above what's going on inside your head and get an aerial view of the spaghetti bowl of jumbled-up unhelpfulness below. Next, take a moment to evaluate each thought, opinion, feeling or idea that's giving you a hard time. Create empathy and further distance by talking about it in the third person to establish that you and it are separate. Assess the worth of each thought, opinion, feeling or idea individually: does it offer a chance of survival in the face of imminent danger? Is it helpful in any other way? Is it worth taking seriously?

Acceptance of thoughts and feelings is optional.

Strategy 4: Breathe (In the Air)

A simple breathing technique to help you relax

In tricky moments when you're feeling tense, grab the earliest opportunity to find somewhere to relax for a few minutes and try this 16-second breathing technique:

Pick out an object with four straight sides, such as a screen, a window, a framed picture or mirror, or a poster of an ad on public transport. Next, follow these simple steps:

1. Breathe in for four seconds as you move your gaze across the top edge of the object from the left-hand corner to the right. Breathe into your belly rather than the top of your lungs, and breathe in through your nose rather than your mouth.

2. As you reach the top-right corner at the end of the four seconds, hold your breath and count to four while rolling your gaze down the object's right-hand side.

3. Breathe out for four seconds while you do the same from right to left across the bottom edge.

4. At the bottom corner, hold your breath, count to four, and move your eyes back to the starting point.

5. Repeat if necessary.

Breathing more slowly is within your control and will physically relax you.

Strategy 5: Ask

Give your Lizard 10 minutes

We know we can't stop Mr Lizard, but we can distract, bore and ignore him, and we can choose whether we listen to him. Ten minutes is usually all it takes to hear him out. When you're feeling low, ask your Lizard what's bothering him.

This idea comes from *The Chimp Paradox*. Dr Peters writes:

"If your Chimp is agitated or upset about something, the first thing it has to do is to release this emotion or opinion. This is called 'Exercising the Chimp'. You must allow it to do this if it is to listen. Allowing the Chimp to express emotion will calm it down and then the Chimp will be able to listen to reason or just go to sleep...most Chimps will take less than 10 minutes to express fears or emotions."

You can either talk to yourself or to someone who won't judge you about your feelings, or it might feel easier to write them down. Devote a few minutes to listening to your Lizard. Ask him what's bothering him. Then ask him why this is a problem for him. Ask him what else is on his mind, and why. Write it all down or just speak.

The point of the exercise is to generate a list of items your Lizard is uncomfortable with. Only then can you establish a way forward based on rational judgement, logic, facts and an understanding of what you can control and what you cannot.

Strategy 6: Release the Pressure

Draw a line and move on

"Don't judge the moment. As soon as you label something as bad, your mind starts to believe it. Instead, be grateful for setbacks." – Jay Shetty, author and former monk

I'd been asked to print a large, important, private spreadsheet. "Try not to look at it," my boss had said.

It was the start of my shift. I'd barely settled into my chair when I could feel my temperature rise and beads of sweat form on my bald head. Others in the office seemed to be much more relaxed as I fumbled my way through printing three illegible versions of the spreadsheet, and one that was just about acceptable.

On to the next task. That, too, seemed harder than it should have been. I couldn't get comfortable at my desk and wanted to start the day again.

My whole 12-hour shift continued in the same vein: unease, discomfort, self-doubt, anxiety. It was exhausting.

Back in my hotel room that night, I sat with a blank page and a pen. I drew a horizontal line across the page, about two thirds of the way down. Above the line, I listed the tasks and emotions I'd struggled with throughout the day. Below it, any positives I could draw from the experience, listening to my internal coach, not the lizardy commentator.

I chose to think constructively. I replaced judgemental comments ("Why did you do that?!") with positive facts ("I've handled tough times before and can do so again.") and 10 things I was grateful for in that moment (my health, the nice room I was staying in, my newly acquired knowledge of spreadsheet printing, and so on).

I realised my thinking throughout that day had been hijacked by my Lizard. I'd forgotten to pause occasionally, breathe deeply and remind myself that I'm capable and in charge.

I learned a lesson: when the day is done, draw a line under the troubling stuff. Write the next day's to-do list and move on. Practise identifying the emotions you feel when you struggle throughout any given day, and devote some time to figuring out why you're feeling them. Don't run away or distract yourself from your emotions. Acknowledge the feeling, sit with the feeling. Name it – 'lonely'? – and it'll dissipate more quickly.

Strategy 7: Feel What You Want

Bring about a sense of calm

"Within our power are opinion, motivation, desire, aversion, and...whatever is of our own doing; not within our power are our body, our property, reputation, office, and... whatever is not of our own doing."

– Epictetus, the Greek Stoic philosopher of the 1st and early 2nd centuries C.E.

When the dorsal side of the vagus nerve reacts to perceived danger, you might feel disconnected and wish to withdraw and isolate yourself. When, on the other hand, you feel safe, grounded and more willing to take risks, this is the ventral vagal state, one of the nervous system's parasympathetic responses.

We can stimulate the vagus nerve and create a sense of calm. The parasympathetic nervous system, the body's 'rest and digest' network, relaxes us after a period of stress by slowing our breathing and heart rate. There are several ways to activate this system and ease anxiety, including:

- Exercise
- Listening to or creating music
- Singing

- Laughter
- Massage
- Spending time in a natural environment (walking barefoot, if possible)
- Spending quality time in good company
- Swimming or showering in cold water
- Creating art
- Engaging in prosody – the patterns of rhythm and sound used in poetry or when reassuring or soothing a young child

A key part of what Djokovic described as "winning that internal fight" is our ability to make positive decisions when it comes to the things within our control:

- Our values, beliefs and worldview
- Our attitudes
- Our thoughts and actions
- How we greet people
- How we treat people

- How we treat ourselves
- What we believe we deserve
- The language we use to talk to ourselves
- The goals we set ourselves
- The people we surround ourselves with
- What we read, watch and listen to
- Our boundaries
- How we manage our time
- How we spend spare time
- Where we place our energy and attention
- How we handle challenges

By that same token, it's also worth remembering that there are things outside our control – things influenced by other people and their relationships, feelings and agendas, and a whole variety of ever-shifting circumstances – that we'd be better placed to try to accept, such as:

- The past
- The future

- Other people's actions, comments, opinions and approval
- How others look after themselves
- Outcomes
- Life's fairness
- Our feelings

But just because we can't *control* our feelings – in that we can't make any sort of guarantee as to how we feel now or will feel later – we can *influence* how we feel, both now and in the future, through our thoughts and actions.

The psychologist Dr Julie Smith explains a simple technique often taught in cognitive behavioural therapy (CBT) that we can use when experiencing difficult feelings.

"Any moment of your life can be broken down into four aspects of your experience:

1. The emotions you're feeling, whether that's happy or sad or anxious or anything else.
2. The thoughts you're experiencing – what's going through your head or how you're talking to yourself. All the things you're focusing on.
3. Your physical sensation – the state of your body.

4. Your behaviour – what you do or don't do.

"We can't directly choose our emotions, we don't have an 'emotion' button we can just press and feel exactly what we want to feel. But we know that those three other aspects of that grid – what you do or don't do, your physical state and your thoughts – impact on how you feel so closely that they're like weaves in a basket. If you start to change those other three, it will have an impact on how you feel and your emotional state. You don't have to be at the mercy of how you're feeling right now. You can make slight shifts in those other things to change how you feel."

Strategy 8: Whatever Gets You Outta the House

Go beyond the front door

Get outdoors. Do something in the open air. Go for a run, get on your bike and ride. Do some gardening, go fishing or join a walking tour and learn about spies or pirates. Do whatever gets you out of the house.

I love the thrill of discovering new music through live performance rather than an algorithm. Seeing Death of Guitar Pop for the first time at the Stone Valley South festival in Hertfordshire, England the day after losing our cherished cat Meg was just what I needed at the time. Hearing great music with friends in an outdoor setting is always a winning combination for me. Simply being there helped.

Schedule an hour or three to enjoy some fresh air. Travel to reach it if you must. Shut the front door behind you and absorb the sweet sensation of breathing beneath the open sky. Make the most of the spring and summer months by getting vitamin D, which the body creates from direct sunlight on the skin when outdoors. Look up and out, not down and inward. Problems feel smaller and you'll gain more perspective with a wider horizon before you. And with that wider horizon, notice the small stuff all around us in nature.

Strategy 9: Walk

Why walking helps

"Our ability to think co-evolved with our ability to walk. It's not surprising, then, to learn that the processes of thinking and walking are deeply integrated.
"The cadence of your walk can influence the inner rhythm of your thoughts and emotions, and vice versa. Therefore, you tend to walk faster if you're excited or angry.
"If you consciously slow down your step, your level of agitation will naturally fall."

– hikeformentalhealth.org

Walking can help to calm the lizard brain and reduce anxiety. When we walk, our eyes continuously shift sideways to provide the brain with ongoing updates about our spatial position. For instance, as you walk and approach a tree, it appears to 'move' relative to your stride, gradually growing larger, signalling your proximity to the tree. This lateral eye movement is known as optic flow, which can deactivate the amygdala – the lizard brain – thereby decreasing the fear response and reducing anxiety.

The act of walking led to the development of EMDR (eye movement desensitisation and reprocessing), an internationally recognised, evidence-based psychological treatment endorsed by the World Health Organisation and the NHS, among other institutions.

Francine Shapiro was an American psychologist who had experienced the diagnosis of her own cancer – and its successful treatment – as well as the death of a younger sibling. Shapiro was interested in physiological and psychological links that could contribute towards physical health.

"One day whilst out walking," Shapiro said, "I noticed some disturbing thoughts in my mind, but also noticed that my eyes were rapidly moving spontaneously back and forth in an upward diagonal. The thoughts disappeared – and yet when I brought them back into my mind their negative charge had greatly reduced."

The EMDR Association UK continues the story:

"Fascinated by this chance discovery Shapiro went on to test this out on over 70 veterans of the Vietnam War so as to create a protocol that could be replicated to decrease anxiety. This protocol became known as Eye Movement Desensitisation (EMD). However, following the evaluation of hundreds of further cases Shapiro noticed that this approach was not just reducing anxiety, it was also helping to change thoughts and the personal meaning of trauma memories. The name of the approach was subsequently changed to Eye Movement Desensitisation & Reprocessing (EMDR). This was a major paradigm shift beyond its original purpose as a treatment for PTSD towards a brand-new psychotherapy."

Strategy 10: Run

My go-to method for head clearance

I'm not a great swimmer. And I failed my cycling proficiency test when I was 12. That's probably why I've never joined my mate Jon to compete in an Ironman event. For me, running is where it's at. I'm not bad at that. It keeps me healthy in mind and body.

Yes, it helps to build strong bones, strengthen muscles, improve cardiovascular fitness and maintain a healthy weight. That's partly why I do it and why I joined a gym (briefly).

But really, I run because it enables me to think less while allowing my mind the freedom to wander where it wants. Ideas and solutions follow, and I always return home feeling better than when I left. And, much as I love music, I prefer to run without it, listening instead to my breathing and steps, and the sounds of nature.

One hour, twice a week, means I'm less likely to swear at strangers under my breath.

Strategy 11: Kill 'Em with Kindness

Be kind to others

"There are three ways to ultimate success. The first way is to be kind. The second way is to be kind. The third way is to be kind." – Henry James, author

Simple things like holding a door open for someone, and bigger acts of generosity such as giving your time and energy, make us, as well as those on the receiving end of such acts, feel better. Acting this way releases oxytocin.

The more oxytocin in our body, the kinder we become, the more we do for others, and the more we *want* to do. We're healthier too, and less likely to become addicted or feed an addiction.

When oxytocin is flowing, we're better equipped to solve problems.

Employ empathy: maybe that person who was nasty is having a bad day, projecting it on to you. But go one step further than simply adjusting your perception of them. Express your compassion out loud. For example, to the lady on the supermarket checkout coming across as rude and moody: "Is your shift ending soon? I hope you get a break." It's her football of worries and issues, not yours, so don't take it on.

Be kind. Feel better.

Strategy 12: Stop

Social media

This one is simple but not necessarily easy.

Facebook, Instagram et al rely on grabbing and keeping our attention in order to make money. And they're very good at it. Social media platforms are designed to take advantage of the way our brains work. They exploit our psychological vulnerabilities. They tap into our core human drives (to acquire, bond, learn, defend and feel) and our FOMO (fear of missing out). If you put your phone down, what will you miss? What will you gain?

We can also influence the algorithms of the feeds we see since Instagram and TikTok will show us more of the types of content we're already looking at and engaging with on those platforms. That gives us some degree of control. Use that control wisely and be intentional about which content you give your time and energy to.

If spending time on social media leaves you feeling worse about yourself and/or regretting how you've wasted precious minutes or hours, stop. Try changing your phone to greyscale or, better still, put it down and occupy your mind and time more positively.

Strategy 13: That's Not My Name

Call it excitement, not nervousness

You might feel nervous when thinking about a future event, or when you're mere moments away from having to do something or go somewhere that fills you with dread, like having to sit in the dentist's chair or enter a new school or workplace for the first time, or perform on a big important stage.

When you're nervous, you might have a pounding heart and sweaty palms, and start predicting what you think is going to happen. Excitement also comes with a pounding heart, sweaty palms and gets us forecasting what we think is going to happen. By consciously reframing an upcoming experience in your head as exciting rather than nerve-wracking, you can approach it more positively.

Practise saying to yourself, "Well, this is exciting", and remind yourself exactly what is exciting about it and why. You're much more likely to have a positive experience this way.

Nervousness, author Simon Sinek suggests, is self-centred:

- "Will they like me?"
- "Am I going to do a good job?"

Excitement, on the other hand, both results from and creates anticipation of connection and generosity:

- "I'm excited to share."
- "I'm excited to give."
- "I'm excited to meet new people and make new friends."

Lots of people find change hard but we can improve our chances of making positive change happen through optimism, focusing on doing our best, and by thinking and acting with generosity and empathy.

Strategy 14: Help

Seek support if and when you need to

"Impostor syndrome doesn't mean others are overestimating you. It's more likely that you're underestimating your potential. "Confidence is often the result of growth, not a cause. Believing in your ability today is less important than believing in your ability to improve tomorrow." – Adam Grant, organisation psychologist and author of *Think Again*

The day before I started my assignment at Wimbledon 2022 as a sub-editor, my friend and career coach Michaela Merten helped me answer some key questions and talk through some aims I had going into the assignment so I could be better prepared psychologically than I had been when I covered the Olympics four months earlier.

The questions I wanted to ask myself and spend time exploring the answers to were:

- How am I feeling going into this event?
- What do I want to experience at this event?
- How do I want to feel when it's over?
- What's been on my mind as the event has drawn closer?

And my aim was:

- To improve my understanding of my past in order to build my future

For a greater sense of security, I wrote my family's names on the back of a photocopy of my event accreditation and put it in my wallet to keep them close at all times.

Through my session with Michaela, I figured out that when the tournament was over I wanted to feel that I'd successfully managed feelings of impostor syndrome and self-doubt, which I'd felt so often when working at previous events.

And what was the thought process I arrived at that helped me work through this imposter syndrome? I figured that every one of the 20,000 accredited media at a summer Olympics had had to start somewhere. They'd all been given a chance at the beginning of their careers, an opportunity. In that sense, we all came from the same place. They were no different from me.

My path to event journalism might have been different from the norm but that was not important. What was important was that I'd stuck with it.

Second-guessing every decision I made along the way was not going to help me with my career. I couldn't predict or control every possible outcome.

Post-Wimbledon, I finally understood that the feelings of uncertainty and doubt I had going into the event are a natural part of growth. They do not signify inevitable failure. They are a precursor to progress and learning.

If you have some serious concerns that are playing on your mind as you approach a key event, worries you're struggling to deal with yourself, you too might benefit from seeking support to work through them. If you need help, you can find links to resources and support – including charities, helplines, books, therapists and the NHS – at the end of the book.

Strategy 15: Morning Glory

What's the story?

Here's an analogy.

Companies can respond to a negative presence on Google by deploying positive search engine optimisation (SEO). By working to replace the bad stories that are showing up on Google's results pages with better ones, organisations can improve their PR and their bottom line.

In practice, that means taking a number of measures, including:

- Publishing a series of positive stories on their website

- Blogging about them, discussing them on social media and promoting them to new and existing audiences

- Optimising their digital properties with keywords and key phrases they'd like to rank for in search engine results pages

- Asking bloggers and other website owners to link to the new stories, which serves as a 'thumbs-up' to Google

What's this got to do with the lizard brain?

Like organisations, we too tell stories about ourselves to ourselves and other people.

What do we mean by stories, in this context? Stories are simply subjective portrayals of events in our lives, how and why certain things are happening or have happened to us, or what we should do in the future. They offer one perspective and, sometimes, they aren't even objectively true.

For example, heading to work at Wimbledon for the first time, I had a few stories running through my head, including:

- "I'm working with a bunch of people who don't know me."

- "I can't let anyone down."

- "I want to be invited back."

These stories made me feel anxious. I needed to change them.

The stories we tell ourselves can portray us in a positive, or a negative, light. They can make us feel relaxed and content, or anxious and on edge.

Like organisations online, we can feel better about ourselves by choosing to tell better stories about ourselves to ourselves and other people, and relegating negative, unhelpful ones.

Take the time to identify the narrative going on inside your head and commit to improving your stories and therefore your worst feelings about yourself.

Here's a suggestion for improving how you think about yourself:

Identify one fact about yourself. An example: you've been picked for a more senior or bigger job than you're used to.

Next, identify one of the stories you tell yourself relating to that fact. It might be: "I shouldn't be here, I don't deserve to be here."

Acknowledge the feeling that fact/story combo (FSC) gives you. Question that feeling. Is it good or bad? Negative or positive? Does it leave you feeling grateful or wanting more? Do you want to keep or change this feeling?

If you want to change the way an FSC is making you feel, consider the likely positive outcomes. The positive outcomes likely to result from the big job, for example, might be personal growth and progress in your career.

The new, positive FSC I constructed for myself as I headed into Wimbledon became:

Fact: I'd been picked for a job I was proud of.

Stories (a.k.a. affirmations in this particular instance. And crucially, all positive, all clearly stated in the present tense and in the first person):

- "I am ready to grow."
- "I allow myself to enjoy my growth."
- "I am the most flexible I can be in this situation."

Whenever you feel doubt or worry, whether it be hidden inside Mr Lizard's jacket pocket or within a beautiful cake made to celebrate your birthday, tell yourself at least one of those new stories, over and over again if you need to.

Strategy 16: Procrastination

When you struggle to get going

Our prefrontal cortex enables us to plan a morning's work. But Mr Lizard, camped out in our limbic system, adds emotion and impulsiveness, becomes distracted, loses focus or seeks perfection. That's the nature of our brains. We confuse, trick and frustrate ourselves. We can reason and we can respond to triggers and threats and temptation. No wonder we procrastinate. Or slow down. Or stop. Or can't get going in the first place.

At such times, we should remember that 'done' is better than 'perfect'.

While some people prefer to work right up against a deadline, feeling it pushes them to do their best work, this approach can also exacerbate problems as it doesn't necessarily allow for issues that hadn't been anticipated or planned for cropping up and demanding immediate attention.

For many, procrastination lies in the difficulty of getting through the surface tension of the task, "the first 10 or 15 minutes," says Dr Piers Steel of the University of Calgary and an expert in procrastination.

I heard Dr Steel being interviewed on the radio when I was avoiding work one morning. The interviewer, newspaper columnist James Marriott, spoke of his personal experience of procrastination being related, in his view, to perfectionism when he opens his laptop to write. Dr Steel, however, pointed out that the link between procrastination and perfectionism, when studied, was found to be "incredibly weak". What's really connected to procrastination, he found, is impulsiveness, driven by our lizard brain. "The more you enjoy the task," he said, "the less hard you have to work to get it away from temptations. At least make your temptations less obvious."

Social media, as we know, is based on temptation: getting and keeping our attention. Dr Steel described social media as "a multi-trillion-dollar platform based upon the top thousand brightest people in the world focusing billion-dollar machines and algorithms directly at your head."

"All your notifications," he said, "your rings, your dings – all these things have the potential to break you from the flow state, and our flow states are gold. That's when you're perfectly engaged in the actual task at hand.

"There's no reason why you should want anything taking you away from that time. You want blocked-out periods of time. And preferably you want it to be a ritual – same time, same day, same routine. And like everything else, it takes about 66 days to get it, for a habit. It's really about getting the habits going."

Help yourself by removing as much room for impulsiveness as possible.

Strategy 17: At The River

Develop good habits

"Every decision I have to make is so much easier down by the river."

– Barry Hearn, a keen angler

Habits are tied very closely to Mr Lizard's way of doing things. The lizard brain can influence the formation of habits through emotional responses. The hippocampus, which is also part of the brain's limbic system and crucial for memory formation and retrieval, helps in linking specific cues or contexts with habitual actions.

When we repeatedly perform an action, especially one that's associated with a reward or relief from discomfort, the brain helps to reinforce that behaviour, helping it form into a habit, by strengthening connections between neurons associated with the behaviour and its outcomes (neurons are nerve cells that carry information between the brain and other parts of the body).

Like Mr Lizard himself, habits can be good or bad for you.

To help form good habits:

- Start small

- Incorporate accountability (when we tell friends or family what we intend to do, we're more likely to do it so we don't feel like we'd lose face in their eyes)

- Track your progress

- Celebrate and reward wins

- Remember why you decided to take this action in the first place

- Have a particular time and place where you can practise these habits regularly

When I'm out running on one of my favourite routes, I'll stop for a few minutes on a bridge which crosses a chalk stream, the river Chess. It's calm there, peaceful and serene, a great place to practise mindfulness. I feel grounded – physically and metaphorically – when I consciously bring my attention to my feet on the earth. I come away with clarity of thought and a renewed ability to find comfort within and outside of myself.

Similarly, one of my favourite places to write is beside a much bigger river: in the Royal Festival Hall's terrace café on London's South Bank. Despite being in the heart of the city, I feel the presence of water there brings a sense of calm.

Mindfulness can take many forms including meditation, gratitude and prayer. What might work for you?

Strategy 18: Reasons to be Cheerful

Be grateful

"Life moves pretty fast. If you don't stop and look around every once in a while you could miss it." – Ferris Bueller, *Ferris Bueller's Day Off*

Have you ever started noticing something more having just learned about it, or soon after that thing has become more relevant to you? Once something catches our attention, we're more likely to notice it again, creating the feeling that it's everywhere. This is known as the frequency illusion, or the Baader-Meinhof phenomenon.

For example, following the death of my mother towards the end of 2023, I would start her car once a week to try to keep the engine working until we found a new owner. With the car now playing a bigger part in my life, I started seeing the same make and model out on the roads, everywhere, even the same colour. They'd always been there but I simply hadn't noticed them before. Now, though, my brain was tuned to recognise them. That's the frequency illusion in action.

The same principle works when we're grateful – and the importance of gratitude on our mental health cannot be overstated. When we're in the habit of reminding ourselves of things we're grateful for, our brains automatically search for more reasons to be cheerful.

10 things

List 10 things you can be grateful for right now, in this moment. A few examples to consider:

1. Your health

2. Your family's health

3. Fresh air to breathe

4. Food on the table

5. A roof over your head

6. The ability and time to exercise

7. Good friends

8. A solid supply of paid work

9. Creative ideas

10. A sense of humour

11. A comfortable bed

12. Your favourite item of clothing

13. Your education

14. Your pet(s)

15. Clean water

16. A well-timed day off

17. Healthcare

18. A good book

19. Your self-awareness

20. A stable internet connection

21. Your favourite food

22. A fun tradition

23. Music

24. Your phone

25. Literacy

26. Your car/bike/scooter

27. Cake

28. Your ability to play a musical instrument

29. Shoes

30. Satnav

31. Free childcare

32. Summer

33. Buddy Holly

34. Salvador Dali

35. Something nice to study

36. Phoning up a buddy

37. Spotify

38. Self-publishing tools

39. AI

40. Good weather

I've found this exercise to be particularly useful in tougher moments.

5,4,3,2,1

Here's another great exercise to get you out of your head and feeling grateful for the wonderful world around you.

Pick out five things you can see right now. What four sounds can you hear? Three things you can touch? Finally, think of two things you can smell and one you can taste.

Relax. Now is all there is. Pause every now and then and recognise the moments when you feel both gratitude and satisfaction. Feeling gratitude and satisfaction at the same time is, I believe, the essence of contentment.

Alright

You're doing OK

Following my work in Beijing at the start of 2022, and by the time my next work event – Wimbledon – rolled around later that year, I'd learned enough insights and strategies to prepare for Rafa, Raducanu and the rest. I knew mindfulness methods. I had affirmations to lean on and breathing techniques to deploy whenever I needed them.

I knew when Mr Lizard was more likely to air an opinion, what triggered him, why he offered the perspectives he did, when to accept them and when (and how) to ignore them. And I realised I already possessed the attitudes, values and beliefs to help maintain brain balance.

The 18 mind management techniques we've explored have helped me and others. I can't guarantee they'll work for you too but they're worth a try should you need something to break a negative pattern, and tell yourself a different story. Practise using them *before* you need them so that using them comes more easily when you do need them.

At Last

A song for resilience

"You can't change the cards you're dealt. What you can do is make the best of the cards. So if someone puts you on a desert island, you make the most of what that island's got to offer." – Barry Hearn, speaking on Desert Island Discs, 25 November 2022

To me, *At Last* represents resilience.

Building resilience doesn't mean life's challenges will simply dry up, nor will things become easier and stay that way. Resilience is the ability to bounce back. Resilience is finding strength and courage when once we might have cracked or wobbled. Stresses will find us. That's life. We just need to be able to identify what's going on, understand why, and manage as best we can with knowledge and self-awareness.

Resilience is consistently working to replace old, unhelpful ways with new, better ways. Resilience is creating new fact/story combos (FSCs). Resilience is creating new neural pathways that will become normal responses when faced with perceived threats.

This song reminds me of when I was on a short break at Wimbledon in 2022, wandering around the grounds.

Competition had started so the public were in. The skies above were blue.

I turned a corner. And there, beneath a balcony at the foot of a few steps and spread out across an open terrace, was a small orchestra. They were playing something I recognised but couldn't immediately name. It didn't matter. It was beautiful. I pulled out my phone and recorded a bit of it.

That moment struck me as one I'd been longing for, a feeling I'd known at many of the previous events I'd worked at. It was happiness, contentment, the combination of satisfaction and gratitude. The song the orchestra was playing was *At Last* by Etta James.

I didn't realise it at the time, but that day marked a profound shift in my mental state.

It was only many months later that I could pinpoint this shift: when I realised I'd not ruminated for days on the kind of minor awkwardness or difficulty I am (and most other people are) confronted with daily – forgetting to thank someone for holding a door, getting a friend's baby's name wrong, not offering to buy someone a drink after they'd bought me one – and which most people give barely a second thought.

But my newfound mental resilience was only truly tested at the end of November 2023, when my lovely mum was diagnosed with acute myeloid leukaemia, and, barely a month later, when she died peacefully at the age of 79.

When she was in hospital, she recalled the words of Marianne Faithfull, when the singer was diagnosed with cancer herself: "I don't want to die – I haven't finished," my mum said. That assessment was pretty accurate: she always had more gardens to visit; art, dance, music and theatre to enjoy; more occasions to celebrate and local walks to explore. She smiled often and like she meant it. We shared values, views, jokes and news. Her influence runs through me like Blackpool runs through a stick of rock.

When she died, I automatically repeated my habit of seeking support, and found loads from family and friends, in song lyrics ("always look on the bright side of life", for example), in books, in articles written by other people who had experienced what I was going through, and in Stoic philosophy. Around that time, I listened to *Be Useful: Seven Tools For Life* by Arnold Schwarzenegger, which is where I came across the Latin phrase amor fati, meaning love of fate, specifically love of *your* fate or one's fate. If we can learn to at least embrace life's challenges – including pain and suffering – suggests this idea, we can find happiness.

I embraced this philosophy, and leaned on it as I managed my emotional response to my mum's death. The amor fati philosophy, which has been linked to the German philosopher Friedrich Nietzsche as well as the Stoic philosopher Epictetus, and Marcus Aurelius, the Roman emperor who was also a Stoic philosopher, encourages creativity, brings people together, teaches us, enriches life and can light a fire in us that inspires positive change. Embracing this idea, I reached the conclusion – just when I needed it – that I loved my life before my mum died because she was in it, and I love my life today *because* she was in it. I'm grateful and I'm happy.

It was a different story when I lost my dad.

He'd died of smoking-related diseases the day before the Beijing 2008 Olympics started. Because of illness, they were the first Olympics he was unable to attend in 40 years. As Reuters' global sports editor, and, later, a consultant to the International Olympic Committee (IOC), the London 2012 Olympic bid team, and the organising committee after London had been awarded the right to host that year's Games, he was admired and respected by many of the world's top sports journalists and administrators, including at least one former president of the IOC. To commemorate his death and reflect this industry-wide respect, a bar was named after him in London 2012's main press centre. Lord Coe attended its opening with us and some of my dad's former colleagues.

When news of his death spread, journalists from all over the world sent warm and loving messages to our family. "He plucked me from news and put me in sport," they said. "He mentored me, he supported me… ."

My parents had divorced when I was about nine, and my dad travelled a great deal for his work. And while he had shown me the art of sub-editing in one brief lesson when I was a teenager, and fuelled my love of sport through his enthusiasm for his work, it felt like there was a void between us, which was partly why my response to his death was very different to how I dealt with my mum's. All I could think at the time of his death was that I had missed out on a lot of the support and care he had shown his staff, colleagues and counterparts. I wanted him to know and notice me like he had them, but felt largely ignored. The physical and emotional distance between us as I'd grown up had left my relationship with him feeling one-way and full of frustration.

Lacking maturity when he died, and the knowledge I've since gained, I struggled to come to terms with the man he was. Although never bitter – my mum wouldn't have allowed that – I felt confused and unhappy: his legacy was inspiring but our father-son connection lacked depth.

Those feelings led to a desire for better, to be gained through knowledge, understanding, self-awareness and clarity. That desire, in turn, signalled the start of the journey to where I am today: enjoying a career which to some extent I owe to my dad's work, and able to draw on much greater mental resilience having made measurable and life-enhancing improvements to the way I think, manage my emotions and handle life's challenges. I've made many of those improvements by following the strategies outlined in this book.

I now place my confidence with care, such as when my brother and I were planning our mum's funeral and I created my own little 'guide to grief', writing affirmations to help me on the day, remembering 'amor fati', and preparing for those moments when I predicted I might crumble. I reminded myself to breathe deeply to relax. In the weeks leading up to the funeral, I ran more often and went for more walks. I tried to stay kind.

Most importantly, then and now, I seek help when I need it, I ask my lizard brain through writing in my current hardback A4 notebook what it is that's causing upset, worry or anxiety, and I focus on gratitude. And then I might listen to The Peace of Mind Playlist.

Resources & further reading

If you're in the UK and you or someone else is in danger, call 999 or go to A&E now. If you need help urgently for your mental health, but it's not an emergency, call the NHS on 111 or visit 111.nhs.uk. Your mental health is as important as your physical health. You will not be wasting anyone's time.

Charities and support

ANDYSMANCLUB - andysmanclub.co.uk

Beacon Domestic Abuse Support Hub (Herts) - oneymca.org/what-we-do/support-advice/beacon-domestic-abuse-support-hub/

Film & TV Charity - filmtvcharity.org.uk

Healthy Young Minds (Lancs/South Cumbria) - healthyyoungmindslsc.co.uk

Hike for Mental Health - ihike.org

Just Drop In (Cheshire East) - justdropin.co.uk

Mend - mend-uk.com

Mental Health Foundation - mentalhealth.org.uk

Mentell - mentell.org.uk

Mind - mind.org.uk

Movember - uk.movember.com

Rethink Mental Illness - rethink.org

Samaritans - samaritans.org

Spoke to a Bloke - spoketoabloke.org

The OLLIE Foundation - theolliefoundation.org

Tonic Music for Mental Health - tonicmusic.co.uk

Visyon (Congleton/Cheshire East) - visyon.org.uk

Coaches & therapists

Saira Hasan - hypno4ladies.com

Michaela Merten - happiness-consulting.co.uk

Ali Moore - bemoore.uk

Owen O'Kane - owenokane.com

Emma Payne - woodland-counselling.co.uk

Alan Whitton - alanwhitton.co.uk

British Association for Counselling and Psychotherapy - bacp.co.uk/search/Therapists

Communities

The Proper Blokes Club - theproperblokesclub.co.uk

Recommended books

Find links to all of them at thepeaceofmindplaylist.com/books

Atomic Habits

How To Be Your Own Therapist

The Big Leap

Switch: How to change things when change is hard

The Chimp Paradox

Fear Less

The War of Art

Quiet: The Power of Introverts in a World That Can't Stop Talking

Think Like a Monk

The Power of Now

Why Has Nobody Told Me This Before?

Mindset: The New Psychology of Success

Be Useful: Seven Tools For Life

Change Your Thinking Change Your Life

For updates on the book, exclusive content and to listen to the playlist, head to thepeaceofmindplaylist.com.

About the Author

Paul Parry is a writer and sub-editor who often works at major international sports events. He loves a good song lyric, the 4/4 time signature, WordPress and Watford FC. He is a partner at Amp Media, the world's greatest content agency serving many major international sports organisations, and an incredibly forgiving driver. *The Peace of Mind Playlist* is his fourth self-published book. His other titles include *Pazzabaijan, Mr Lizard,* and *Working Remotely – How to promote your internet-based business.* He is often on his laptop and always at paulparry.com.

Acknowledgements

In creating this book, there are lots of people I need to thank. I should probably start by thanking my wife, Shoelace, and our beautiful daughters for making me want to be a decent human being – and for making me the occasional morning coffee.

To my brother, Dan, thank you for helping to knock my first draft into something grown-ups might actually get something from. Huge thanks too to my sister Hannah for her unwavering support and encouragement, the incomparable Luke Norman and Nick Moore, who make working at Amp Media such a pleasure. Thanks to my fun and thoroughly professional event colleagues, and my mates, all of whom act as my therapists from time to time. Huge gratitude of course goes to all the brilliant authors, speakers, athletes and healthcare professionals whose work or words I and so many others have leaned on.

To Susan Bush, thank you for helping me deeply consider my aims with this book; to Rachel Kenny, thank you for your peerless editing and support; and thanks to Kate Lamb for having the courage to speak out about mental health in the context of working at a large international sports event. Further hat tips go to Jonathan Cooksley for always being there with his boundless creativity, unique artistic capability and solid perspective on business; to the marketing geniuses Jacob Rickard and Ryan Hills; Jon Jackson, Richard Jones, Stuart Gill and Death of Guitar Pop's Silky, who all gave their time so generously to help me produce better work. Huge thanks must go to Tony Conroy for so generously donating his supreme subbing skills to improve my marketing copy, and, like Keith Moore, Eusébio Galvão and Roddie McVake, for taking the time to listen when things got a bit on top for me during the Beijing 2022 Olympic Winter Games. Everyone needs at least one good listener in their life. And to the qualified practitioners who so unselfishly gave me a slice of their wisdom, Emma Payne, Ali Moore, Alan Whitton and Micheala Merten, thank you. Thanks too to Dr David Cox, whose reassurance that the science information in this book wasn't made up or gleaned from the back of a box of Frosties was the stuff of dreams, and to Graham Nye and Sharon & Andy Joynson, who've all given me unrivalled support in producing this book.

And of course to all the musicians and lyricists – not just those featured in this book – whose work has kept me sane my whole life, you make the world go round.

For book updates, premium content and exclusive offers,
join my mailing list at TPoMP.com

Printed in Dunstable, United Kingdom

74158761R00087